WEIGHTLIFTING PROGRAMMING
A WINNING COACH'S GUIDE

BOB TAKANO

WEIGHTLIFTING PROGRAMMING
A WINNING COACH'S GUIDE

BOB TAKANO

Catalyst Athletics, Inc.

*To my loving wife Marta, who made the writing of
this book a reality, my stepson Freddy, and all the
lifters I've coached over the years.*

CONTENTS

FOREWORD
BY HARVEY NEWTON

The exciting and demanding Olympic sport of weightlifting has experienced a renewed interest in America over the past decade or so. This is partially due to the strong support for weightlifting-type training by organizations such as the National Strength and Conditioning Association and the Collegiate Strength and Conditioning Coaches Association. It is also partially a result of CrossFit, the popular form of physical training that embraces weightlifting's key competitive movements, the snatch and the clean & jerk.

As with most sports, getting better at weightlifting requires proper coaching. Successful coaching of weightlifting requires proficiency in at least three domains: developing optimal exercise technique, creating and implementing proper program planning, and appropriate knowledge and skill directed toward achieving success on the competitive platform.

Most newcomers to weightlifting coaching correctly focus their energies on observing, understanding, and instructing the technical intricacies of our challenging lifts. The novice coach quickly realizes that successful competition coaching comes over time and cannot be rushed. Lost in the middle of this sequence is how to design and implement sound training programs. Lacking an understanding of scientific training principles or the ability to design proper training protocols severely limits one's ability to succeed.

With *Weightlifting Programming: A Winning Coach's Guide*, Bob Takano, a senior international coach and lifelong educator, provides the road map for weightlifting success. Bob is a longtime friend and coaching colleague, one I trust to correctly and intelligently get the word out to present and future weightlifting coaches about the right way to train.

Initially, Bob and I obtained our coaching knowledge through similar methods, including learning from others, digesting foreign coaching publications, and a good deal of trial and error methods applied to junior lifters. Long before I got to know "T", I was influenced by his regular writings in the former *International Olympic Lifter* journal. His original column, Exercise of the Month, which evolved into Takanotes, was always a highlight, and illustrated not only his insights into technique and training concepts, but also showcased him as an excellent writer.

As USA Weightlifting's first national coach, I invited Bob to attend camps and courses at the U.S. Olympic Training Center in Colorado Springs so I could watch firsthand his coaching methods. I also had the pleasure to coach internationally a number of Bob's lifters, especially USA Olympian Albert Hood. Young Albert demonstrated the results of Bob's excellent coaching at the junior world championships and the 1984 Olympic Games.

In the late 1980s, I organized USAW's first attempts at coaches' education. Gene Baker, our National Coaching Coordinator at the time, designed and executed three manuals dealing with technique, general physical preparation, and program planning, along with two videotapes. What proved fascinating was the runaway success of the third manual, *Training Program Design*.

Gene and I quickly concluded that most coaches want a cookbook approach to training; that is, "Show me someone else's program and I'll implement it." This is certainly the easiest way to access a training program, albeit perhaps not the proper program for a particular weightlifter. Few seemed inclined to learn *how* to develop a program or to go through the sometime laborious effort of doing the math involved. Similarly, at the NSCA I found far too many certified strength and conditioning specialists (CSCS) basically clueless as to how to design an annual plan.

Some readers will take the same approach after reading *Weightlifting Programming: A Winning Coach's Guide*. Bob even mentions "... stealing training programs ..." as an early coaching tactic. But he goes on to clearly state that to be successful, one must eventually delve into and utilize the volumes of valuable information provided in this one-of-a-kind book.

Weightlifting coaching is a challenge, one not easily mastered. Shortcuts, such as following the latest Internet fad workout, seldom pay off, particularly in terms of reaching the Olympic level. As a reader, you have in your hands a fantastic resource of proven training methods designed to optimize weightlifting performance. Cherish the experience!

—*Harvey Newton, newton-sports.com*

SECTION A
INTRODUCTION

There is currently more interest in participation in weightlifting and performing the Olympic lifts in the United States than at any other time in history. The membership of USA Weightlifting, the national governing body of the sport, is larger than it has ever been. The sales of bars suitable for performing the snatch and clean & jerk and rubber bumper plates are far in excess of any previous figures. Weightlifting shoes have become relatively easy to purchase over the internet and in some cases there are stores that carry them. More people than ever before have taken and passed the beginning level USAW Coaching Certification (USAW L1), and the CrossFit Olympic Lifting Certification is booked as much as a year in advance.

University Strength and Conditioning facilities have replaced weight machines with platforms and Olympic bars and bumpers. The interest in performing snatches and cleans & jerks and their derivative movements is growing, and so is the thirst for training knowledge. Private gym owners and instructors, professional strength and conditioning coaches, physical education teachers and other workers within the athletic and fitness industries are anxious to learn the best methods for coaching and performing the Olympic lifts. Aside from attending clinics and seminars that range widely in quality of information, seekers may find the pathway to coaching competency twisting and full of dead ends.

As might be expected there is a relatively large number of people offering clinics and seminars. Many of them have dubious credentials and minimal experience. More than a few of them are charging excessively for attendance and the information disseminated is frequently sketchy, incomplete or highly unrepresentative of the well-organized body of knowledge involved in training weightlifting athletes.

Much of this confusion is due to the fact that the United States has no standardized credentialing or licensing program for athletic coaches. Furthermore, there is no organization that is concerned with certifying the authenticity or validity of information sources. Most true professions have a national body that licenses or certifies individuals as to their competencies and ability to disseminate legitimate information from an acknowledged body of information. And although there are thousands of professional coaches in this country, there is no national certifying body. Subsequently determining the qualifications of a coach or instructor can be difficult or highly challenging.

Part of this is due to the fact that the United States has never fully appreciated the scope of the education that is required of a professional coach. Whereas nations that take sports seriously offer and provide demanding coaching curricula and degrees, the USA has never seen the need to impose rigorous academic standards for coaching candidates even in the sports that are immensely popular.

Currently there is little chance that a coaching credential will be required in any sport any time soon. Its very existence would nullify the employment of thousands of coaches, and then recertifying them in any meaningful way would be an immense task. Some grandfathering would probably be the best solution while requiring newcomers to become fully certified.

While most beginning weightlifting coaches need to master the essentials of teaching proper technique, those that intend to move forward with their coaching education must master the science and art of program planning to ensure the continued progress of their athletes. Currently the bulk of coaching education for weightlifting in this country is directed at the process of mastering technique coaching.

This will only occupy part of an athlete's career—a very small part. The rest of the career will be taken up with training. The skillful planning of that training will determine the continued progress of the athlete. Currently there is very little available to coaches wanting to master the process of program design.

It is with the thought of fulfilling this need that has provided the impetus for the writing of this book.

—Bob Takano, August 3, 2011

CHAPTER 1
THE PROBLEM, THE DILEMMA

You want to coach weightlifters, and you've done everything you can to advance your knowledge. You've taken the CrossFit Olympic Lifting Certification, and passed the USA Weightlifting Sports Performance Coach Certification. You've even started coaching some juniors and entered them in competitions and the results were pretty rewarding. What next?

As it currently stands, the quest for knowledge in weightlifting in the United States is not a well-directed path. Any aspiring weightlifting coach is probably facing a daunting task. What I'd like to do with this book is remove some of the mystery from the process of program planning, a critical component of the list of coaching functions.

Most coaches are going to figure out how to coach technique, and a large percentage are finding out that it's not as challenging as some "experts" in the strength and conditioning world would have you believe. I've personally seen some coaches who've taken either of the aforementioned certifications and shortly thereafter begin developing athletes with fundamentally sound technique that will only get better with more training.

After this short initial education on coaching technique, the coach is then faced with the task of writing training programs that will ensure progress to the point where the athlete's potential is realized.

Most exercise science majors in college physical education, exercise science and sport science departments are required to complete courses in anatomy, physiology and kinesiology. No argument there. But there is very little information available as to how to put that knowledge to use in a meaningful way for a weightlifting coach or for a coach in very many other sports for that matter.

The National Strength and Conditioning Association (NSCA) has adopted the credo "Bridging the Gap" to bring about some application of scientific principles to the actual coaching of athletes. Unfortunately this goal is still a ways from being reached since there isn't enough common background between sport scientists and sport coaches.

The gap does not even begin to address the issues of pedagogy, sports psychology, competition management or any of a large number of other problems that enter into the equation of becoming an effective coach.

This leaves the coach being forced to learn the many aspects of the art and science of coaching without any established curriculum, and without any established sport institute or university to provide or at least anoint the most effective course of learning.

At this point the best prescription I could provide would be to participate in the sport of weightlifting for a prolonged period of time in order to understand the feelings involved with training and competing. One of the tasks of a coach is to be able to describe "feelings" to athletes, and this is accomplished most readily by those individuals who have felt them and put some thought into the methods of conveying the concepts.

If during this participation, the athlete/prospective coach can be coached by an accomplished coach, the chances of succeeding as a coach are enhanced. Watching the process in action is one of the best ways to understand the many facets of the task. Watching a variety of coaches carry out their duties is also extremely helpful.

Those of us who chose teaching as a profession got to watch at least seven elementary teachers, at least 18 middle school teachers and at least 24 high school teachers do their jobs. At some point we probably took note of the techniques that worked and which ones should have been avoided. A major part of coaching is teaching and the same approach can be applied. A mentorship under the supervision of an accomplished coach is probably the most significant educational experience that an aspiring coach can undertake in the path of coaching development.

Of course during all this time, some time needs to be spent learning and understanding the scientific principles involved with the process of athlete development. There are a number of formal curricula available, but much of what needs to be learned can be done on an individual basis by those of a studious nature.

It is at this point that the coaching development process can quickly level off if not stall altogether. The next logical step would be to study and assimilate the available translations of Russian texts. While these are full of valuable information, they can be cumbersome and are not necessarily organized to be understood by those with less than a university background in sport science with a specialization in coaching weightlifting.

Keeping this in mind, I've moved forward with this book in an attempt to try to provide a source of information for one of the key functions of the weightlifting coach. The material has been derived from a wide variety of sources over many years. The least of these has not been the tremendous number of coaching hours in the gym that has produced a large number of highly successful weightlifters. All of this is being put forward in an attempt to provide a valuable step for those aspiring to become weightlifting coaches.

Until the infrastructure of the sport is upgraded, this will have to serve as just another small step in the pathway.

SECTION B
SPORTS PHYSIOLOGY AND
THE HUMAN ORGANISM

This section concerns itself with the raw material from which coaches must draw performance. It is concerned with the human species, and how genetic material is dispersed and manifested. Only through understanding the processes through which the genetic material manifests itself in the functioning body can coaches concern themselves with altering and refining these processes in order to bring about superior athletic performance.

As a secondary science teacher with forty years of experience, I am well aware that Americans are, as a culture, remarkably science-phobic. I have a well thought out, though not quite scientific, understanding of the phenomenon. This phobia should not be allowed to provide a major impediment to a comprehension of the process that I've dubbed *protoplasmic engineering*. That is what you are doing when you plan training in order to bring about an improvement in performance through a remodeling of the tissue.

You, as an aspiring coach, must understand that you are embarking on a process of altering the functional capabilities of a medium—protoplasm, or living tissue. Just as with any creative process, the creator must have some understanding of the medium. If you are a musician, it would make sense to improve your understanding of the functional nature of air. If you are a photographer, you would undoubtedly have to spend some effort in studying light. To be a weightlifting coach, you must have an understanding of protoplasm. It is no longer possible to elicit a change in the body of an elite athlete or even a mediocre athlete by considering it to be little more than a black box.

I also have some interest in the human species and how its evolution has affected its participation in sports. We are currently in an interesting period in the short history of the modern form of our species. Due to the nature of the plasticity of our brains, our capacity to manipulate tools, and our propensity for finding solutions through the formation of societal groupings, we have created civilized environments that have altered the selection process of our species. This section is therefore focused on what a human is from a biological/physiological standpoint.

Chapter 2 is dedicated to the last 50,000 years or so of human history. I find this interesting and something that needs to be taken into consideration by any individual or group interested in designing a program that will select and develop individuals to a very high level of accomplishment. This certainly pertains to fields of endeavor that extend well beyond just weightlifting. The migration patterns of humans have had a profound effect upon how elite programs are organized to select and develop talent. A few of the national governing bodies of Olympic sports have focused on which factors are to be considered as they develop their athletes. Most have not.

Many of the readers of this book will someday move into positions of governance and administration of sports programs and it is with some optimism that I include this chapter so that those readers will begin to develop some appreciation for the anthropological factors that affect international sport.

Chapter 3 covers the well-worn topic of homeostasis. Most coaches have some understanding of the phenomenon, but most American coaches have not become adequately familiar with the process as it pertains to athletic development. Although I cover the topic in a very general way, my hope is that this will provide some appreciation for the subject and pique the curiosity of the developing coach.

It is not uncommon for many instructors and coaches within the physical training fields in this country to become fixated on a very narrow range of topics, and expect them to apply to all too many situations. Little effort is given to understanding the broad processes that are taking place in the development of the athletic body. The weightlifting coach must understand these broad processes and their application to the design of training.

This short two-chapter section is an effort to provide coaches with some basic concepts that can affect and influence their thinking toward the task of program design.

CHAPTER 2
THE HUMAN SPECIES

My approach to coaching sports has always been based on an understanding of my medium. In this case it is human protoplasm. I need to know quite a bit about how it works, how it can be changed and how it got to be the way it is in its present state. This may not be of great immediate interest to a lot of beginning coaches, but I think that at some point you, as a coach, will have to spend some time thinking about this topic.

First of all, humans are a rather unique species of large mammal. We are the only mammals who are habitually upright walkers. That requires us to have a larger base in order to balance on two feet. This has been accomplished by our primate predecessors by developing a foot where the heel is in contact with the ground. Consequently, not all of us are comfortable pushing up on to the ball of the foot in order to generate explosive power with the legs and hips. This is something we, as coaches, have to deal with on a consistent basis.

Another point that makes weightlifting a unique human sport is that we have shoulders with a tremendous range of mobility. Thanks to our brachiating primate ancestors, we can hold our arms vertically overhead, and thanks to our habitually upright walking, we can comfortably support weights overhead. We also have opposable thumbs that we can use to form a hook grip. Finally, we have a grotesquely large brain. It has in fact grown from about 450 cm^3 to about 1,500 cm^3 in the short evolutionary time span of about 5,000,000 years. This fact has enabled us to effectively ponder and implement the process of athletic development as no other species ever has.

I enjoy coaching humans.

Global Migration

Although there is some debate among paleoanthropologists as to the approximate date of the exodus of *Homo sapiens* from Africa, the migration that led to the populating of the planet probably took place between 50,000 and 60,000 years ago. From Africa, the human species became the largest and only mammalian species to walk and/or sail to every habitable landmass on the planet.

Because of the exceptionally large human brain, the prehensile fingers and opposable thumbs, the development of speech, the non-specialized digestive system and the structure of human social groups, the migrating humans were able to inhabit an incredibly wide variety of environments. From the Arctic Circle to tropical rainforests to the most arid deserts, humans established viable habitations on every continent with the exception of Antarctica.

Out of Africa

Those first migrations had human populations leaving Africa undoubtedly in waves of varying sizes. Obviously the first land mass occupied was Eurasia, followed by Australia and the North and South American continents. By 14,000 years ago, *Homo sapiens* was living on every habitable environment on the planet. The study of mitochondrial DNA (or mDNA) points to an African origin, as does the study of the development of languages. Both studies indicate greater and greater variation as the studied populations are found to have originated farther and farther from Africa.

It is remarkable for such a large species to have adapted so quickly to such a wide range of habitats and environments. It is indicative of the tremendous plasticity of the adaptational abilities of our species as well as non-genetic factors playing a part. In short, the development of our brains has allowed us to solve survival problems without having to develop any protein-based solutions through structures and enzymes.

From a morphological standpoint, humans must be considered generalists. They are not possessed of great physical strength or especially great endurance. Without tools, they are not especially effective consumers of plant materials or killers of prey. The digestive system is neither as long as would be expected of a pure herbivore, nor as short as is typical of carnivores needing to avoid putrefaction in the lower gastrointestinal tract. The array of digestive enzymes secreted by humans favor an omnivorous diet.

Local Adaptation

As previously stated, by 14,000 years ago or thereabouts, humans had occupied a wide variety of environments. Each environment provided different factors that could affect the survival rates of its human inhabitants and subsequently the frequency of certain alleles (alternative form of a gene) within the population. This had the effect of favoring certain phenotypic characteristics over others.

Local Environments

The local environments that exist around the planet that were occupied by early *Homo sapiens* were determined by the usual assortment of factors: average daily temperatures, photoperiodicity, soil content, annual average rainful, native plants and animals, communicable diseases and the vectors, terrain, and numerous others. They were responsible for shaping the local genome (the collection of the genes of the local human population), by altering the ratios of alleles. This in essence is microevolution: the changing of allelic ratios within a local population and not the entire species.

This had the effect of changing the phenotypes (physical representation of the genes) of local populations. Certain phenotypic characteristics would provide a differential in either survival or reproductive rates or both, and thus would change the survivability of the local population within the local context. Thus a tall, thin equatorial resident adapted to losing heat would quickly experience hypothermia if dropped into the polar conditions of a population adapted to a much more frigid environment.

These reconstitutions of the local gene pools by the environments took place over a relatively short span of time in geological terms, and as such the Earth was populated by a variety of difference local types up until very recent times when rapid mass transcontinental migration became a reality.

Genetic Isolation

The movement of genetic material is often not significant if only single individuals periodically leave one isolated group and join another. Most groups remain relatively isolated, and although at any time they could co-mingle DNA with other isolated groups and still produce viable, fertile offspring, certain physical traits and capabilities that were genetically-based developed in some isolated populations. Some of these traits would have provided an advantage in certain types of athletic competitions, while others would have been a definite hindrance.

Much of the genetic makeup of these isolated populations is still in existence in many of the 200+ member nations of the International Olympic Committee. As a result, some of these nations will excel in certain events and not perform as well in others. The nations that have a greater chance of succeeding in the wide panorama of Olympic sports are those with a wide variety of phenotypes from which to draw.

Genetic Recombination

Within the biological sciences community, genetic recombination refers to the pairing of alleles through the union of sperm and egg between a male and female. In this discussion, I am using it to refer to the rejoining and recombining of isolated gene pools that were developed from that initial worldwide migration.

At one point there was a single male and single female that gave birth to the first true *Homo sapiens*, and that produced a limited gene pool. The aforementioned worldwide migration produced a change in the genome through mutations and local isolation.

What must be intriguing to coaches is how these local populations can re-unite and form new combinations that result in individuals that are best suited for a particular physical activity.

As a paradigm, we can consider the breeding of domestic animals. It is not uncommon for breeders to combine two breeds to form a third with a combination of desirable characteristics of the parent breeds. Coaches cannot regulate such breeding in humans, but we are constantly on the lookout for that rare individual who has inherited desirable characteristics from both parents that provide an uncommon advantage in a particular sport.

Civilization and Cities

The concept of civilization and cities has much to do with the development of specialized athletes. One of the hallmarks of civilization is the increased productivity over a hunter-gatherer or even pastoral type of existence. This would then lead to taxation so that the wealth could be redistributed and used to sponsor individuals who perform specific tasks that are beneficial to the culture as a whole, but not necessarily associated with the survival of the group.

Coaches and athletes fall into the category of those who benefit from the development of civilization. Per se, they do nothing to aid in the survival of the group, but if supported they can achieve results that are important to the culture.

Cities are where these cultural activities can take place most effectively, as they will reach the greatest number of people. Cities, because of their ability to generate wealth, will also attract a large number of people. Modern cities attract descendents from these local isolated populations and thus provide the environment for mass genetic recombination to take place.

Mass Continental Travel

During the 20th century, mass transcontinental travel and hence migration became easily accessible to a significant percentage of the world's populations. National governmental control notwithstanding, the world's local populations were able to leave the local environments that did so much to shape their genetic constituencies and venture out into cities that were populated by other immigrant groups.

Large ships, trains and now airplanes have contributed to this mass transporting of DNA around the globe. Most of the world's population now lives in cities, and although there are abundant cultural taboos against mating with members of other immigrant groups, miscegenation is relatively common in cities.

This means that there is a constant, ongoing process that will randomly lead to individuals who are more likely to be more genetically suited for a given sport than their predecessors. The chances of finding an ideal physical type for a particular sport are much greater in a city than in a more isolated setting where there is a great deal more genetic isolation and less gene flow into and out of the population.

The Near Perfect Genotype

Some sports are heavily talent-dependent, while others are less reliant on talent, but more dependent on training and development. Some sports require a large variety of skills, and those that can master the greatest percentage of those skills can overcome more talented athletes with less skill development. Other sports have metabolic requirements that are spread across the three energy pathways, all of which can be enhanced to a degree, and therefore success can be accessed by the athlete willing to spend the most effort in intelligent development of the three pathways.

The sport of weightlifting favors the mesomorphic somatotype, with a well-developed motor cortex, and a high percentage of muscle fibers that are capable of high contractile rates. One issue that is infrequently discussed is the fact that the distance between the inner collars places a limitation on the length of the arms and the width of the shoulders in such a manner that there is a height limit on weightlifters. One method of finding individuals of this favorable type is to recruit from localized gene pools in which those phenotypic characteristics are prevalent. Otherwise the best-suited phenotypes must be sought out amidst larger gene pools.

Variety of Sports

There are 28 different sports contested in the Summer Olympics, and some of them favor very specific physical traits or combinations of physical traits.

Variety of Somatotypes and Phenotypes

Short of island nations, countries are geopolitical entities with boundary lines often drawn by mutual agreement between adjoining nations. As such, they do not necessarily serve to provide physical isolation of the genetic material within the boundaries. There are within each nation a variety of somatotypes and phenotypes. The representation of nations at the Olympics and World Championships represents a somewhat contrived template on the population genetics involved. What is therefore represented is a combination of genetic factors and sociopolitical infrastructure. This represents more variables and makes the results all the more interesting.

The successful weightlifting nations are those that can identify the talent, entice it to participate, and groom it properly while supporting it. In order to do this successfully, the anthropological factors must be considered.

One issue that has arisen within the 21st century has been the introduction of women's weightlifting in the Olympic Games. This means that there will be official government sponsorship of the sport in the over 180 member nations of the IWF. More than that, however, is the fact that in most countries, male and female weightlifters will be using the same training facilities and undoubtedly interpersonal relationships will develop. I don't want to sound like a "master race" guy, but if highly selected men and women reproduce, the chances of talented individuals being generated are heightened considerably. This will facilitate the talent identification process considerably.

All of these many factors will come into play as the sport of weightlifting progresses through the 21st century.

CHAPTER 3
HOMEOSTASIS

All species on this planet have some capacity for homeostasis, the ability to return the organism to a state of constancy or stasis. This state may also be considered the one that uses the least amount of energy. Organisms by nature are always having to deal with the issue of entropy, the tendency of matter in the universe to behave in chaotic, non-random patterns.

In order for an organism to function, a certain amount of energy must be devoted to maintaining molecules in certain structures or certain pathways or behaviors. With energy at somewhat of a premium, organisms tend to use it in the most economical ways just to maintain life processes.

As an example, humans normally synthesize red blood cells that transport oxygen around the body to the cells. Those cells have a normal life span of 100 to 120 days. At that point, they die and their materials are recycled by macrophages and new red blood cells are synthesized by the bone marrow to replace them. This synthesis is triggered by the secretion of the hormone erythropoietin by the kidneys. The synthesis requires energy expenditure to assemble the new cells.

If the oxygenation of the tissues is adequate, the body continues to secrete erythropoietin at a consistent rate, resulting in the synthesis of red blood cells. If the general activity levels of the organism drop, creating a lowered need for oxygen, the body will respond by secreting less erythropoietin (The process of synthesizing erythropoietin always requires energy.), subsequently saving the energy that would be needed to synthesize red blood cells.

So homeostasis is the sum total of the body's physiological processes to maintain a stable internal environment. This concept is the most important one to understand in the planning of training of athletes.

If we consider weightlifting training to cause a disruption of homeostasis, the body will attempt to adapt to the stress of the training and return the body to a lower resting energy state.

General Adaptation Syndrome

The General Adaptation Syndrome (GAS) was first described by the Canadian physiologist Hans Selye in his 1956 book, *The Stress of Life*. My physiology professor, Dr. Patrick Wells, assigned this reading to my class of sophomore biology majors and I am forever indebted to him for that. Little did I suspect at the time that it would prepare me for a weightlifting coaching career.

Selye was the first to describe non-specific stress upon organisms and the physiological response to that stress. He explained how an organism subjected to stress, a factor that upset the normal functioning of the physiology, would respond by making adaptations, either temporary or long term to prevent the stress from further disruption of homeostasis.

An understanding of the GAS is essential in the planning of programming for the training of weightlifters.

Stressors

Stressors are factors that cause a disruption of the physiology of the organism. To return to the original example of the synthesis of red blood cells mentioned earlier, a stressor might be a prolonged lack of sufficient oxygen or hypoxia due to moving to an increased altitude or exercise that creates oxygen demand beyond that which can be supplied by the individual's existing physiology. Or it could be the opposite, an increase in oxygen availability due to spending time in a hyperbaric chamber. Both of these types of stressors would affect the synthesis of red blood cells, which would be the adaptation made by the organism.

In terms of training weightlifters, a eu-stressor is a factor that brings about a desired change. A dis-stressor is one that brings about an undesired or deleterious change—sickness or injury. Frequently, a eu-stressor can become a dis-stressor if it is administered too frequently or in excessive amounts.

Eu-Stressors A eu-stressor for a weightlifter is one of the factors that is generated by the training program. It can be the intensity, load, volume or frequency. At the beginning of a training macrocycle, the athlete's endocrine glands are secreting appropriate amounts of the various hormones to maintain good general health. As the macrocycle proceeds, the training load or volume may cause the endocrines to exceed their normal secretory capacities.

If adaptation takes place within a reasonable period of time, the training factors have functioned as eu-stressors.

Dis-stressors If the training factors accumulate their effects in such a way that the athlete becomes severely overtrained, injured or catches a cold, then they have become dis-stressors. They have exceeded the adaptational capacities of the weightlifter, and will not generate the adaptations that will lead to an enhanced performance beyond the capacities of the lifter at the beginning of the macrocycle.

The same factor, if imposed in too great a dosage or too frequently, might initially start out as a eu-stressor and then become a dis-stressor.

One of the functions of program design is to attempt to impose eu-stressors to the appropriate levels before they become dis-stressors. Sometimes the reasonable limit is exceeded, but this is to be expected when both the coach and the athletes are competitive individuals and anxious to achieve the greatest gains possible.

Adaptation

Adaptation is the process of making changes in the structure and functioning of the weightlifter's body in response to the eu-stressors. These changes are initiated by the hormones secreted by the endocrines and carried out by the protein anabolizing mechanisms of the cells.

They can be assisted by the provision of appropriate substances, and by restoration methods that must be regularly incorporated in order to raise the adaptational threshold of the organism. The topic of restoration will be covered in Chaper 15. This concept is a new frontier in athlete preparation and one that is still ripe for investigation.

The term applied to the final adaptation to a major training cycle is *supercompensation*. This describes the condition in which the tissues and functional capability of the physiology have been changed to accommodate the latest types and quantities of stressors.

Tissue Remodeling

Tissue remodeling is the process of both changing the structure of the cells and the relative proportions of specific cells and their compositional relationships within the organs of the athlete. Many weightlifting enthusiasts focus too much attention on the remodeling of the muscles. Although muscles are of great importance, the tissues of the tendons, ligaments, bones, nerves, endocrines and digestive organs must also be modified in a competitive weightlifter.

If the training of muscles is not accompanied by sufficient stresses on the connective tissues (bones, ligaments, tendons), they will not be remodeled and strengthen, resulting in injuries. Since the ligaments and tendons are avascular, they tend not to heal very rapidly, and an injury to these structures can inhibit the progress of training and subsequently development.

It is quite obvious that bones must be strengthened in order to bear the great loads imposed upon them by the sport of weightlifting. The stresses placed on bones will result in them incorporating more calcium salts into the matrix (non-living portion) of the bones. This affects bone density and is reflected in the weight of bones.

Protein Synthesis

The process of protein synthesis (or anabolism) is the method by which genes are expressed. The information (nucleotide sequence) in a particular segment of a DNA molecule (the exon) is transferred to a messenger RNA molecule that takes that information out of the nucleus of a cell to the cytoplasm where amino acids are assembled into protein molecules.

The specific sequence of amino acids in a protein molecule represents the organismic "talent" of an athlete.

Two individuals may have the same nucleotide sequences to synthesize a given protein, but the frequency with which those sequences are activated may determine the final outcome in terms of performance or ability. So just the presence of a particular gene may not be the only factor in determining athletic success. This may help to explain why there may be a great disparity between the siblings of talented parents.

Structural Proteins

Most protoplasm is composed of water. In humans, the amount is roughly 70 percent. Of the dry weight of protoplasm, 95 percent is protein. It's not hard, then, to understand that the form taken by a human body is largely the result of the structure imposed by structural proteins; otherwise a human body would be little differentiated from a puddle of water.

The structural protein that is of the greatest interest to weightlifting coaches are the contractile proteins actin and myosin. The thicker myosin filaments have extruding structures call S1 subunits that move actin filaments along the length of the myosin. This action produces contractile or shortening forces along the length of a muscle.

The amount of force generated by a muscle is determined by the number and arrangement of the actin and myosin myofilaments, their ergogenic support matrix and how many of them can be stimulated simultaneously.

Enzymes

Enzymes are protein molecules that facilitate very specific biochemical reactions both within and without cells. Enzymes have very specific structures, and each enzyme can only function on a very specific substrate or reactant. Although the molecules of the reactants in a chemical reaction may freely coexist without interacting, the activation energy needed to initiate the reaction can be excessively high and in fact potentially damaging to the cell. This is the safety mechanism to prevent these reactions from taking place without appropriate signaling from the organism. The function of an enzyme is to lower that activation energy so that the reaction can proceed forward. Each enzyme can only perform this lowering for a specific reaction.

The reactions can be either anabolic, in which a larger molecule is assembled from smaller molecules, or catabolic, in which a larger molecule is broken down into smaller molecules.

An enzyme will continue to perform its function until it is in turn broken down by a specific enzyme. Thus for each chemical reaction in the body, there is an enzyme that controls its commencement and another enzyme to cause it to cease.

Hormone Secretion and Receptor Sites

Hormones are lipid-based or protein-based molecules that are either secreted into the bloodstream by the endocrine glands or affect cells that are local to the secretory cells. The hormones secreted into the bloodstream are responsible for global effects (their effects are not localized) throughout the body. They flow through the body and attach themselves to target cells by binding to receptor sites on the cell membranes. Receptor sites, made up of proteins or glycoproteins, are specific to each hormone, so that a testosterone molecule, for example, will not bind to a receptor site for insulin.

Receptor sites also vary in number and concentration on different cells. It is not known how receptor sites come to exist on the cell membrane. The effects of certain hormones could be enhanced if the development of receptor sites could be stimulated by training factors. They may well already be, but research has yet to verify this.

When a steroid (lipid-based) hormone binds to a cell, it initiates protein synthesis by certain genes in the nucleus. This causes an increase in the synthesis of that particular protein and the functionality of the cell is then enhanced. A catecholamine (water-based hormone) will bind to a receptor site and then initiate metabolic changes within the cell. This will cause an activation or de-activation of the specific function of the cell.

One of the significant adaptations that must be evoked by the manipulation of the training load is for the endocrine glands to increase their capacities to secrete hormones. During the preparation mesocycles, the training load will cause a hypersecretion of hormones. This will continue until the endocrines enhance their capacities to secrete. When the training load is dropped down during the pre-competition mesocycle, the endocrines are still secreting at elevated levels and the circulating hormone levels are enhanced and thus initiating a greater restoration of the muscles and the other relevant structures.

It is the direct goal of the training program design to initiate this hormonal/endocrine gland response that will lead to the remodeling of the tissues, and hence the production of a higher functioning athletic physique.

SECTION C
WEIGHTLIFTING TRAINING

The early weightlifting competitions were focused on determining which athletes were the strongest. The first officially recorded weightlifting competition took place in Vienna in 1896. Not surprisingly, the best results were achieved by butchers. Butchering large animals requires a great deal of physical strength and only those possessed of great natural strength could even begin to do the work. Unquestionably, the hard physical labor helped to make them even stronger.

Throughout the late 19th and early 20th century, athletes were being trained to get stronger, and this could be verified by the invention of the plate-loading barbell by a Russian physical culture professor in 1896. This replaced the shot-loading barbell, which was a device for resistance training that varied the resistance through the addition or removal of lead shot in the globes at either end of the implement.

The plate-loading barbell made it possible to standardize the lifts that were used in competition and undoubtedly led to the formation of the International Weightlifting Federation (Federacion Internacionale Halterophile et Culturiste) in 1905. It also provided the opportunity for athletes to train with heavier and heavier weights without the inconvenience of loading and unloading shot, and increased the total possible weight that could be loaded on a barbell.

The focus of the various national groups was to not only select the strongest athletes, but to develop the most effective technique of lifting the weights and to train for that task. Thus was born the concept of weightlifting training with the barbell as a standardized implement.

Centuries-old data indicates that humans had developed training methodologies dating back to ancient times as long ago as the Egyptian empire. The implements, however, varied from civilization to civilization and it was not until after the industrial revolution of the 19th century that the thought of the standardization of sports apparatus began to take shape.

With the advent of the plate-loading barbell, equipment could be standardized and subsequently competitive events could be defined and standardized as well with the possibility of accurate record keeping becoming a reality. Unquestionably, the development of science also pointed toward the standardization of sporting events in order to acquire comparable knowledge of human physical capacities.

It is therefore not surprising that the development of the barbell, the standardization of weightlifting competition and the rise of scientific investigation all occurred almost concurrently within a few decades in Europe. As a result, Europe has since dominated international weightlifting save for the decade after World War II (when Europe was recovering) until recently, when the rise of the Asian nations has provided a meaningful threat to that dominance.

The nature of the training, the sport itself and the implements involved have made the training of weightlifters a particularly attractive topic for research by sport scientists. The fact that the training takes place in a relatively small amount of space, and that the overwhelming majority of the training is conducted in easily measurable units, has made the study of that training especially attractive to the researchers.

That quantitative aspect has facilitated the studies of periodization and the adaptational characteristics of athletes. Once understood, much of those general concepts could then be used to explain training phenomena in other endeavors. Accordingly, weightlifting is very fundamental sport in the sport science universe.

With the larger concepts having been articulated and assimilated, most of the progress in the world competitions will result from the best implementation of these concepts. Infrastructure, talent identification, pedagogy, nutrition, sports medicine and restoration are now the areas of challenge for the world's training systems. This type of overarching approach will be necessary for those national federations concerned with raising the world standards.

At the heart of it all, however, is the design of training programs and the degree to which they are modified for each talented individual. In the best systems in the world, the number of athletes per coach is limited to four. This allows the coach to get to know each athlete's training and performance parameters intimately and to make the appropriate modifications in the training programs. The coach who can make these modifications most deftly will be the one who produces the weightlifters with the best performances. The first step in mastering this modification process is an understanding of the principles behind training program design.

CHAPTER 4
A BRIEF HISTORY OF
WEIGHTLIFTING TRAINING

The true development of weightlifting training didn't take hold until national governments with financial resources took an interest in sports. The prestige bestowed upon sports by the Olympic Games made it the focus of nations wishing to propagandize the supposed superiority of their political systems. The first nation to take a serious interest was Nazi Germany, which allocated resources to sports science and the selection and training of athletes.

Although German weightlifters did well prior to World War II, no startling breakthroughs in training methodology came forth from their research, although there is some indication that the early research into tissue-building drugs and nervous system stimulants may have had their origin under the Third Reich.

It was not until after World War II when the Soviets saw the propaganda value of the Games that sport science began in earnest. At the direction of the Soviet government, extremely bright students were funneled into the Sports Institutes of the Eastern bloc to begin research on sports training methodologies and the best ways to develop Olympic level athletes.

Sports were fully launched as a major part of the Big Red Propaganda Machine. Culturally, the Eastern European nations are geared toward educating and developing exceptional individuals. This applies to athletes, coaches and scholars.

This is a major difference from American culture where the emphasis is on manufacturing and marketing goods. Consequently different sports develop at different rates in the two camps.

Those sports that are less equipment/technology dependent with little commercial potential thrived in the Eastern Bloc, while those sports that had great dependence on expensive equipment and facilities better suited American culture.

Most of the Olympic sports have little commercial potential or spectator appeal and as such they cannot generate sufficient funding or even *raison d'etre*. Without sufficient funding for facilities, athlete salaries or coaching salaries, these sports cannot exist even as subjects of applied research in the universities.

Defining The Sport

The original Olympic weightlifting competition had no weight classes and the contest lifts were the two-hand and one-hand lifts overhead. As stated previously, there was probably very little in the way of training, but rather the sport became a matter of selecting the strongest athletes. Weightlifting was not included in the 1904, 1908 and 1912 Games, but was reinstated in 1920 under the organization of the International Weightlifting

Federation.

The 1920 Olympics were the first Games to feature the two lifts that still remain as competitive events, the snatch and the clean & jerk. At that time the one-arm snatch, the one-arm clean & jerk and two hands press were also a part of the competitive program.

From the first official world championships held in 1905 until 1972 when the current two-lift format was adopted, the sport was in the process of defining itself. Except for changes in bodyweight classes and the inclusion of the women into the Olympic Games in 2000, the competitive program has remained in stasis for a considerable period. There are periodic calls for change in the events contested, but the IWF has maintained the existing standard. The only foreseeable change might be the addition of a bodyweight class.

1924

The 1924 Paris Olympics were the last Olympics to have five lifts contested in the weightlifting competition. The one-arm snatch and one-arm clean & jerk were eliminated from the competitive program from that point forward. This shortened competition and obviously changed the approach to training.

1972

The 1972 Munich Olympics saw the last major world competition in which the two-hands press was contested. Some felt that the officiating of the press was becoming too inconsistent and was failing to maintain a standard. Competitions were often overly long because of the number of lifts, and the potential for back injuries was increasing with the weights being lifted. These weights were approaching and in some cases exceeding the weights lifted in the clean & jerk.

Furthermore the most athletic aspect of the press was the clean. The increased number of cleans also raised the average intensity and had an effect on the speed of movement of the athlete. In an effort to streamline the sport and emphasize the athleticism of the competitors, the IWF Congress voted to eliminate the press. I was present in Munich for that vote. As soon as it became final, I promptly mailed my training partners in Los Angeles so that they could stop training for the press.

1992

After several years of doping positives, the Olympics reached a low point for weightlifting in 1988 when several lifters were found to test positive for performance enhancing drugs or illegal diuretics. That, coupled with the furor surrounding sprinter Ben Johnson's positive after obliterating the men's 100 meter sprint record, caused the IOC to severely rebuke those federations that were not taking sufficient measures to curb the problem.

One of the sticky issues that confronted the International Weightlifting Federation (IWF) was the problem of world records that had been established under the obsolete and questionable doping control standards of previous years. The existing records were very high, apparently the result of unregulated sports doping. Therefore the IWF decided to make 1992 the last year for the existing bodyweight classes, and all the existing records would subsequently be retired.

Thus 1993 began with new weight classes for both male and female competitors. The new men's classes were 54, 59, 64, 70, 76, 83, 91, 99, 108 and 108+ kg. The new women's classes were 46, 50, 54, 59, 64, 70, 76, 83 and 83+ kg. The number of classes was unchanged with 10 for men and 9 for women. The women's program was still not included in the Olympic Games. This is significant, as for most countries, this is the trigger for funding to be provided. Minimum standards were established for new records in order to prevent an overflow of world record claims.

1996

This marked the last historical change in the rules that govern the competitive nature of the sport. In 1996, the IOC agreed to include the women in the weightlifting competition in the 2000 Games. Women's weightlifting world championships had been conducted since 1987, that first one being in the United States. 2000 would mark the debut of women's weightlifting in the Games. The IOC, however, was only willing to increase the number of gold medals given to the sport of weightlifting from 10 to 15. This meant another revision of the classes. It was decided to designate 8 classes for men and 7 classes for women.

The classes for men would now be 56, 62, 69, 77, 85, 94, 105, and 105+ kg. The classes for women would now be 48, 53, 58, 63, 69, 75 and 75+ kg. These classes took effect on January 1, 1998.

There has been some criticism of the women's classes as there is quite a gap between the 75 kg limit and the winners of the 75+ kg class. This eliminates a certain percentage of the female population from competing on a fair basis. There is a large enough percentage of women who stand in the height range where they would not be effective at clean & jerks at 75 kg bodyweight, but would not be able to perform athletically at 95 or more kg bodyweight and be competitive with the true behemoths in the 75+ kg class.

As we have seen, the rules of a sport periodically change under review, so there is some hope that the women's classes might someday be changed to provide a truer representation of women's heights than they currently do.

Post World War II and Sports Science

World War II begat the Cold War period when the two predominant ideologies of Democracy and Communism stood at odds with each other. The development of readily available television, the launching of communication satellites and the rise in prestige of the Olympic Games all led to a bloom in the development of Sports Science and its application to athletic competition.

The sudden acceptance of the Olympic Games as a legitimate test of the world's athletes soon came to be portrayed by the Soviet bloc as an opportunity to tout the superiority of the Communist system. Once the Soviets had recovered from the War in terms of human and economic resources, the Big Red Sports machine was put into motion.

Sports Institutes were constructed in all of the Eastern Bloc countries and efforts were made to funnel some of the brightest students into the Physical Culture programs to become physical education instructors, coaches and sports scientists. Daunting admission exams testing proficiency in math and science had been put into place to ensure that only the brightest could become sports professionals. The first two years of college were filled with math and science courses to insure that there would be a common basis of understanding, a common body of knowledge, and a common means of interpreting empirical information between the members of the three professions.

Furthermore, the scientists had access to the coaches and athletes. This provided a fertile testing ground for new techniques, new technologies and new training approaches. Accurate data could be recorded and analyzed to allow coaches and sports medicine professionals to take the best approaches toward developing top-level athletes. Because of the common educational background, the communication lines between the various professionals were open and available.

The Solidification of Training Knowledge

This time period, from the end of World War II until the fall of communism in 1989, produced a body of sports science knowledge that has yet to be matched. No other nation or group of nations in the world is as committed to sports science research as was the Soviet bloc. Much of that knowledge has become available to the rest of the world since 1989, as the many top coaches gainfully employed by the "Big Red Machine" were dismissed as the new emerging republics temporarily downsized their sports programs.

For example I've heard that Bulgaria, which had 85 full time weightlifting coaches prior to 1989, downsized briefly to only 2 after the death of Communism. Those coaches fled the country and many have been employed by other nations as the paradigm for the development of weightlifters has slowly shifted away from the old amateur rules that prevailed under Avery Brundage.

The knowledge possessed by those coaches is now being used around the globe, and nations that had previously been minor lights in the weightlifting sky have now begun to find their athletes on the medal podium with greater frequency.

Even before the break-up, publications of training articles had been leaving the Iron Curtain with some regularity and due to the translation efforts of several dedicated scholars such as Andrew Charniga and Michael Yessis, fans of Soviet training who had a fairly thorough knowledge of the methodologies. Apparently after a certain familiarity with our non-system was acquired, the Soviets did not feel threatened by free world lifting nations, and were not so possessive of their knowledge.

What has been difficult to learn about and discern is the sports pharmacology and the means of restoration. Because of the longstanding ban against performance enhancing drugs, the hesitation to discuss the pharmacology is understandable. Restoration after hard training that enables the athlete to train with greater load and intensity more frequently is apparently not of very great interest to many coaches in America, but it is a major part of the reason why many athletes around the world are able to train harder than their American counterparts. Restoration, I believe, is the next great frontier in sports training knowledge.

Part of the problem for the lack of interest in restorative means is largely due to the American fascination with labor saving devices and substances. We are not especially interested in learning about new methodologies that would allow us to work harder.

There is apparently enough of the information for athlete preparation available, but the world is in need of solidification and integration of all this knowledge. The solidification is yet to be done.

I don't believe that most of the purveyors of training knowledge are necessarily attempting to conceal their methodologies, since the sale of knowledge is more of a marketing concept consistent with American capitalism. In my experience most of the foreign coaches were perfectly willing to impart knowledge. In fact it is the implementation of training knowledge that is really the determining factor. Effective coaches figure out implementation most effectively. Moreover they understood that information must be accompanied by pedagogical training and some mentorship in order to be fully effective.

This book is being written with the intent of providing some information. It is up to the individual to seek paths that will enable implementation and the oversight of effective mentors.

CHAPTER 5
GENERAL CONCEPTS

In order to master the art and science of training weightlifters, a coach must understand some broad concepts that will enable him or her to properly implement and tinker with the training variables in order to reach the optimal results.

There must be an understanding of the developmental and maturation processes of the physical body and the psychological state. In spite of cultural bias to the contrary in the United States, weightlifting is a sport best performed by adolescents and young adults. There are appropriate aspects of training that must be implemented within the proper windows of development in order to reach the full genetic potential of the individual athlete.

The planning of training must take into consideration the timeline of development and the fact that smaller athletes will mature at a more rapid rate than larger athletes. Smaller athletes have a greater capacity for restoration, and that is a significant factor in the design and planning of training.

The coach must also understand the proper amount of emphasis that must be placed on training, psychological development, skill development, nutrition and restoration, for the misplacement of emphasis will also fail to yield optimal results.

These many factors and conditions must be balanced in the mind of the coach while planning and implementing training if there is to be a harmonious development of the organism and ultimately an optimal performance level on the competitive platform.

The PASM

The Process of Acquiring Sports Mastery (PASM) was a concept introduced by former world superheavyweight champion and Soviet national coach Alexei Medvedyev. He graphically portrayed the development of the young organism in such a manner that the appropriate timing of various aspects of developmental enhancement would lead to an optimal development of the athlete.

His concept of implementation of motor skill development coincided with the development of the motor cortex in the young athlete, as did his concept of implementation of general physical preparation coincide with the somatic development. Significant strength training was introduced at a time when it would coincide with sexual maturation so that the hormonal secretion would be in greatest demand during the time of greatest secretory activity. All of these factors were integrated and introduced at the proper time and in the proper dosages to ensure the full development and lengthy career of the weightlifter. Under his watch, the Soviets produced a profound number of champion weightlifters, many of them with long and distinguished careers.

We periodically find out about overzealous parents who are implementing excessive amounts of strength training to pre-pubertal children with the concept in mind that this will lead to many appearances on the medal stand, when in fact the timing is wrong. This strength training is being introduced at a time when the motor skills and athletic coordination should be developing, so consequently those aspects of development are minimized and the full athletic potential is not reached.

Others may want to start weightlifting when they are in their late teens and have never been introduced to proper athletic training during the formative years. Many of these adolescents are enamored of attaining great physical strength, but do not comprehend that physical strength is only a portion of the developmental needs of a weightlifter. They too will fail to reach their optimal athletic condition for weightlifting.

Medvedyev's writings and publications have become revered pieces of training literature, and could well serve as a textbook for anyone wishing to undertake the education necessary to become a weightlifting coach.

I must forewarn coaches wishing to undertake the study of the Soviet generated material. Although they are translated into English, there is some familiarity with the idioms, cultural idiosyncrasies and philosophies that must be mastered to truly understand some of the concepts.

Growth and Maturation of the Organism

Human beings take a long time to reach full physical maturity for an organism of their size. Usually small mammals reach physical maturity in a relatively short period of time. Mice, for example, are mature at several months of age. Horses on the other hand reach physical maturity in the third to fourth years of life. Small humans may be physically mature at 14 years, while larger individuals may not reach full physical development until 23 or 24 years of age.

Part of this lag in development is due to the time necessary for the human brain to develop within the human social context. Consequently, the physical development takes a considerable amount of time as well, as the motor coordination is tied into the maturation of the motor cortex of the brain. There is a certain amount of plasticity to the motor development of pre-adolescent humans. Even those youngsters blessed with excellent motor skills can refine them even further with appropriate training during the maturation process. This is what takes place in the training of gymnasts, acrobats, dancers and divers who start out at a very high level and then, through long and regular training, attain skills levels that are absolutely unattainable by the majority of athletes.

With the inception of the Youth Olympic Games, the School-Age World Championships and the Junior World Championships, the impetus to find and develop young weightlifters has increased. The top weightlifting nations are finding athletes succeeding with exceptional weights because they are mastering proficient technique at a very early age. These accomplishments are demonstrating that previous concepts of athletic development were underestimating the capacities of talented youngsters. The future results of these youngsters as they develop will provide us with a more accurate perspective on this issue of young athlete development.

Consequently various physical aspects of development mature over a wide variety of times. This needs to be comprehended and coaches must not necessarily use the anomalous development of prodigies, although in sports we are always looking for prodigies.

There are appropriate developmental activities for athletes during the pre-pubertal stages. These include motor development, intellectual development, and improvement of both global and local circulation. Appropriate competitive attitudes may also be fostered during this period. Emphasis of these areas during this pre-pubertal stage will lead to less time emphasizing them during the latter stages.

The Proper Age Range

When I visited Bulgaria in 1989 before the fall of the Evil Empire, I was able to speak with some of the members of the national coaching staff. They were rather upset that the Sports Ministry allowed figure skating to select athletes for training at age 6, but that weightlifting would have to wait until youngsters were age 12.

Their argument was that a great deal of the athletic talent was siphoned off to figure skating and other high motor-learning dependent sports before weightlifting had a chance to select. I could see their point, but I think we all realized that motor learning prodigies needed to be introduced to a sport like figure skating at an early age if they were to have a solid shot at becoming a world-class competitor.

In Bulgaria and the rest of the Eastern bloc, young prodigies were enrolled in sport schools where they spent their mornings in classroom activities, and their afternoons engaged in age-appropriate athletic training activities. A weightlifter selected at an early age would have had to spend time doing very little specific weightlifting work and more general physical preparation activities. These did not necessarily require a sport school, but a sport school situation would allow for monitoring of development as well as the development of the athletic psyche.

If you had a child who had some physical talent or the right bloodlines for being a weightlifter, those pre-pubertal years would need to be spent in general physical preparation if he or she were to eventually develop into a top weightlifter. Basic physical skills such as running, jumping, throwing, swimming and competing in games would all serve the athlete best at that point in the development.

General Physical Preparation

The reasons to include general physical preparation early in the development of the athlete are several and of considerable importance. They are all not just physical, but also involve psychological and emotional maturation emphases.

When I coach an athlete coming to me during early adolescence, I can easily determine whether or not there has been a history of proper, balanced childhood athletic development. An athlete at this point demonstrates advanced coordination, balanced physical development, emotional maturity toward the training process, and great energy reserves.

Youngsters who have access to physical activity at an early age have had an extensive amount of experience learning how to "drive the car" that is their bodies. Neural connections have been established that may not develop so thoroughly at later stages of development. Local muscle endurance, and respiratory capacities are also enhanced by vigorous physical activity during the pre-adolescent period.

All of this will result in an ability to deal more effectively with the rigors of weightlifting training as that development continues through adolescence. Because of the proper synergy in muscular development there will be fewer injuries and there will be continuous strength increases and technical acquisition. The improved circulatory capacities will enable faster restoration, as will the enhanced respiratory capacities.

Another aspect that is not often considered is the development of the psyche for the athletic lifestyle and the capacity to perform on demand. A youngster entering puberty with a background in maintaining some daily regimen, receiving coaching advice, competing successfully and performing on demand will have a significant advantage over others lacking these experiences.

All of this GPP must be maintained and enhanced during the early days of weightlifting training. The days during which there is no weight room training, and even in addition to weightlifting sessions, GPP sessions can be conducted. They can be composed of running and jumping games (basketball, volleyball, team handball, football), track and field events, gymnastics activities and grappling. Swimming in moderate amounts is also an effective restoration modality that can also be included in a GPP regimen.

One of the most helpful modalities of GPP for weightlifters is the use of jumping exercises. Consecutive, sequential jumping from a quarter squat to a full squat depth in sequences of three to five jumps employ the stretch shortening cycle in a manner that is helpful for the generation of explosive force of the legs and hips. These types of jumping activities can be done with both feet, and when the athlete becomes stronger they can be performed on a single leg with a partner running alongside holding the off leg.

I've also had a great deal of success having my athletes jump up a staircase that was 16 steps high. They would jump up taking three steps at a time. This was performed for three to five sets from two to three times per week. When they became stronger, they would go up four steps at a time. Some of the more advanced athletes would jump up 5 stairs at a time.

When an athlete could negotiate the staircase jumping five stairs in each jump, I would add three sets of jumps performed three stairs at a time on a single leg. Jumping up staircases forces the jumping to be more vertical and since there is very little drop, the impact on the joints is minimized.

For purposes of improving motor unit recruitment I would program this stair jumping alternating with sets of back or front squats. This was especially helpful in developing the explosive leg strength of my lifters.

For athletes who have trained for at least 2 years, depth jumps can be employed. They are of the greatest value when the athletes can squat double bodyweight. They can be performed from a height as great as 2 meters, but the height should not be so great that it forces the heels to touch the ground upon landing. The focus of this type of training is to minimize the ground contact time while attempting to jump as high as possible upon landing. 15 to 20 jumps can be performed per session, and should not be done more frequently than 7 to 10 days.

Obviously very heavy athletes should avoid jumping from great heights in order to spare the joints from excess trauma.

Of course, all of these activities must be coordinated so as not to conflict with the goals of each weightlifting training session. The amount of GPP is gradually reduced as the athlete proceeds through the various class rankings.

Other Developmental Considerations

Technical training for weightlifting could be introduced during late childhood/early adolescence using just a dowel or PVC pipe, and most athletic prodigies would have little trouble learning the technicalities of the snatch and clean & jerk just by watching a competent practitioner perform the movements. The less talented motor learners will need some technical coaching.

And of course since I was a school teacher, I would also have to put a major emphasis on age appropriate classroom learning activities. I was once told by a Bulgarian weightlifting coach, Angel Angelov, who was coaching the Mexican national team during the late 1970s, that if two athletes were equal in ability, the more intelligent one would be the one preferred. Keep in mind that this was coming from a Communist coach who was used to exerting more control over his athletes' lives than we Americans could ever hope to, and yet he felt that the more intelligent athlete would be able to make the best choices.

What we would now have is an athlete at the onset of puberty with excellent motor skills, the ability to perform technically sound lifts with light weights, the capacity to undertake larger than average training loads and the intelligence to make sound decisions about training and life. At this point, the coach could begin the process of developing greater training capacity specific to the sport of weightlifting in the body of the athlete.

From this point on we would expect to see the athlete undertaking a greater and greater training load each year until reaching his or her late 20s, when the body's own restoration capacities would begin to wind down and we would have to back off on the dosage. By this time, the athlete would have been expected to develop competitive efficiencies to compensate for the drop off in restoration capacities.

After the age of 30, most weightlifters who have had a serious career that began in the early teens will be dealing with the many nagging injuries that are typical of a lengthy career, and the healing of those injuries would inhibit the full training of the athlete over prolonged periods. This is demonstrated by the fact that the vast majority of Olympic medalists are in their 20s, and only occasionally do we find one in his or her 30s. This is becoming more so as the sport has become more developed.

The Bodyweight Issue

The empirical results indicate that there is an appropriate bodyweight range for a weightlifter's height. Younger weightlifters, especially in the heavier classes, tend to gain significant muscular bodyweight over the competitive career and move up one, two or even more classes. The ratio of strength of the body overall is not in direct relationship with the bodyweight.

The issue of the appropriate bodyweight for height can be explained by comparing two lifters with identical bodyweights, but one is significantly shorter than the other. If the percentages of muscular bodyweight are identical, the taller one is attempting to move longer limbs with the same amount of muscular mass. While attachment points can explain some of this disparity, if the height difference is significant, it cannot make up for the fact that greater muscular force must be generated to move the longer lever.

The smaller the organism, the greater the relative strength of the weightlifter. As an example, the first athlete to snatch double bodyweight was Yoshinobu Miyake in the

60 kg class in the early 1960s. It is now commonplace for top international lifters in that bodyweight range to snatch double bodyweight. The first triple bodyweight clean & jerk was performed by a 60 kg lifter, Stepan Topurov in 1983. A number of athletes in that bodyweight range and lower have exceeded the triple bodyweight mark.

At the other end of the scale, the heaviest snatch ever lifted is 216 kg by Antonio Krastev, who performed that lift in 1986. His bodyweight was approximately 160 kg, meaning he snatched 1.34% of his bodyweight, a far cry from double. The all-time world record clean & jerk for superheavyweights is 266 kg, performed by a 152 kg Leonid Taranenko for a percentage of 1.75—not even double bodyweight.

So lifters become more inefficient as they get larger. They also do relatively worse in the clean & jerk if they are not at the proper bodyweight for their height. Coaches and athletes need to realize that it is not the bodyweight per se, but the ratio of bodyweight to height that determines proficiency in lifting.

One of the ratios that needs to be considered is the ratio of snatch to clean & jerk. For a lifter who is well balanced, training properly and lifting in the proper weight class for his or her height, the snatch will fall in the range of 78-82% of the clean & jerk. All things being equal, if a lifter is too light for his or her height, the ratio will exceed 82% by two or more percentage points. This range was derived from data taken before the current drug testing technology was in place. As we move forward it appears as though the snatch will be a higher percentage of the clean & jerk largely due to less performance enhancing drug usage. Although these ranges probably hold true for the women, as well, the short period of time during which women could establish a base level from 1987 to 1992 probably does not provide us sufficient data for an appropriate comparison.

As a lifter matures and gets older, the ability to train heavy enough frequently enough diminishes, and this has the greatest effect on the clean & jerk. Subsequently the athlete needs to gain weight in order to keep the clean & jerk at the proper level.

The calculations in Table 5.1 for ideal height ranges for top international class male lifters were calculated using linear interpolation of Robert Roman's data by Shaun LeConte. These figures should be considered guidelines, but I feel they are entirely appropriate.

Weight Class	Height Range
56 kg	149 ± 3 cm
62 kg	156.33 ± 2.5 cm
69 kg	161.75 ± 2 cm
77 kg	165 ± 2 cm
85 kg	169 ± 2 cm
94 kg	172.5 ± 2 cm
105 kg	176 ± 2 cm
+105 kg	186 ± 6 cm

Table 5.1 Height Ranges for Male Weight Classes

Height ranges for female lifters were one of the parameters undertaken for Leslie Musser's Master's Thesis. The subjects were the competitors at the 2009 Pan American Weightlifting Championships and the figures should stand as representative ranges for top-level international lifters. The +75 Kg class was not measured. (Table 5.2)

Weight Class	Minimum	Maximum	Mean	SD
48 kg	139.00 cm	152.50 cm	148.00 cm	4.96 cm
53 kg	149.00 cm	155.50 cm	152.80 cm	2.75 cm
58 kg	150.50 cm	159.00 cm	154.33 cm	3.09 cm
63 kg	150.00 cm	162.00 cm	157.17 cm	4.57 cm
69 kg	152.50 cm	164.00 cm	158.42 cm	3.99 cm
75 kg	159.00 cm	167.30 cm	163.26 cm	3.63 cm

Table 5.2 Height Ranges for Female Weight Classes

It is especially common among many adolescents to fail to comprehend some of these concepts, but the coach should begin the process of educating lifters as to the optimal ultimate bodyweight class. This can be effected through presenting the heights of the top competitors and matching them with their lifts and the ratio of snatch to clean & jerk.

Another set of model height indices for weightlifters was developed by A.V. Chernyak of the Soviet Union in 1978 for the men's classes at that time. His work delineates the appropriate heights for the various Ranking Classes (These classes are discussed in Chapter 6) to provide some guidelines for the development of the bodyweight through career. (Table 5.3)

Qualification	Range	52	56	60	67.5	75	82.5	90	110	+110
Novice	Minimum	153	156	163	168	174	179	181	182	--
Class 3	Maximum	158	163	168	173	179	184	186	187	--
Class 2, 1	Minimum	150	155	160	165	170	175	177	178	--
	Maximum	155	160	165	170	175	180	183	183	--
CMS-MS	Minimum	148	151	157	162	166	170	174	178	--
	Maximum	152	156	162	167	171	175	179	183	--
MS-MSIC	Minimum	144	148	155	159	163	167	171	176	183
	Maximum	146	150	157	161	165	169	173	178	188
World Record Holders	Minimum	144	148	154	159	163	167	171	176	183
	Maximum	145	149	155	160	164	168	172	177	189

Table 5.3 Model Height Indices for male weightlifting classes and bodyweights
(Height in cm; weight in kg)

WEIGHTLIFTING PROGRAMMING

In 1978, the 100 kg class was only a year old and there might not have been sufficient data to derive figures for that class.

Although this table reflects the pre-1993 weight classes, the trends are obvious. I believe that one of the great values of this table is that it provides a direction for the developing athlete and the coach with respect to the appropriate bodyweight. All too often I have seen talented athletes with great potential intentionally forced to lose bodyweight and lift in an improper weight class simply because it would increase the standing of the athlete in national events. If this practice is maintained for extensive periods, it will have a limiting effect on the long-term development of the athlete. In the United States, there is a dearth of competitors in the lighter bodyweight classes and so a talented athlete can often lose weight and lift winning weights. This sometimes goes on for much longer periods than are appropriate for the overall development of the athlete.

The information in this table or one adjusted for the current weight classes will do much to point the coach and athlete toward the ultimate appropriate bodyweight.

A thorough understanding of these general concepts will allow the coach to thoughtfully implement the training information that is presented in the following chapters.

CHAPTER 6
THE ORGANIZATION OF
WEIGHTLIFTING TRAINING

The training of weightlifters is organized into specific phases that correspond with the development and maturation of the organization. There is some variation with respect to the chronological age of the athlete as shorter athletes tend to mature at an earlier age than taller athletes, and there are, of course, genetic issues that must be taken into consideration. These issues include the muscular somatotype of the individual, specific digestive efficiencies, protein metabolism, and hormonal profile. The general plan is geared toward working with talented youngsters with the foundation being established during pre-adolescence. Athletes entering the sport after puberty are much less likely to achieve their ultimate genetic potential.

During the pre-adolescent period, prospective weightlifters should be involved in a fair amount of general physical preparation in order to develop athletic qualities, and develop the support systems that will enable demanding training and sufficient restoration to take place at later stages of training. The lungs and breathing apparatus, local circulation and motor capacities should be addressed during this time. Competitive games practiced during this period will also aid in the development of the athlete's psyche. All of this preparation is appropriate for many sports, so there is little need for specialization. The practicing of proper technique with light bars is also helpful.

During puberty the general physical preparation is diminished and more weightlifting and strength building exercises become more essential. The body is in a state of hormonal transition that is beneficial for the development of strength, and the development of the skeleton and connective structures. The implementation of heavier weights in the performance of the specific weightlifting movements will serve to develop a harmonious physical structure for the future performance of the snatch and clean & jerk.

Shortly thereafter, some attention must be given to the increase in load in order that the body will develop a greater capacity to perform demanding training and then restore more rapidly. At this point the technique should be highly refined, and attention will be given to developing strength and speed-strength characteristics. The athlete should also be developing proper habits of hygiene and lifestyle and learning how to perform properly in competitive situations.

The next phase should be the period during which the athlete is fully developed in terms of motor, physiological and psychological qualities. The training will be most demanding in its impact on the physiology and the highest results should be realized. As this phase nears its conclusion, the training must accommodate the aging physiology and the training must become more efficient, but the athlete should have a greater competitive aplomb that will help in achieving exceptional results that are consistent with the genetics.

The Classification System

Weightlifting results are easily measured in kilograms, and it is this objectivity that has attracted so much interest from the sports science community. Consequently, because weightlifting competition is conducted by dividing competitors into bodyweight classes, it is easily possible to calculate standards of excellence based on hard quantitative data.

Just such a system was developed in Eastern Europe called the classification system. In this system, there are six levels in ascending order: Class 3, Class 2, Class 1, Candidate for Master of Sport, Master of Sport and International (or Merited) Master of Sport. Each bodyweight class is assigned a total for each level. (See Tables 6.1 and 6.2)

This system allows athletes to be grouped by proficiency levels, and to assign appropriate developmental training protocols. Empirical evidence supports the concept that optimal results are attained at the end of a career if the appropriate training is assigned at each level.

It also allows competitions to be designated for particular levels so that more objective conclusions can be made as to the proficiency levels of the developing weightlifters. It is especially effective in those programs that have a large population of lifters. The effectiveness of the program can be determined by the movement of athletes through the various classes. Tables 6.1 and 6.2 provide the qualification figures for men and women.

Weight Class	Titles and Levels								
	Adult Males						Boys 11-16 years		
	MMS	MS	CMS	I	II	III	I-Youth	II-Youth	III-Youth
32 Kg			85	75	65	60	50	45	40
34 Kg			95	80	70	65	55	50	45
38 Kg			105	95	80	70	65	55	50
42 Kg			120	105	95	80	70	65	60
46 Kg		160	135	120	105	90	85	75	70
50 Kg		180	155	135	120	105	90	85	75
56 Kg	255	205	175	155	135	120	105	95	85
62 Kg	285	230	195	175	155	130	120	105	95
69 Kg	320	255	220	190	170	145	130	115	100
77 Kg	350	280	240	210	185	160	140	125	110
85 Kg	365	295	255	225	195	170	145	130	115
94 Kg	385	310	265	235	205	175	155	135	120
105 Kg	400	320	275	240	215	185	160	140	125
105 + Kg	415	325	280	245	220	190	165	145	130

Table 6.1 Male Weightlifting Classification

Weight Class	Titles and Levels								
	Adult Women						Girls 11-16 years		
	MMS	MS	CMS	I	II	III	I-Youth	II-Youth	III-Youth
32 Kg			75	65	55	50	45	40	35
36 Kg			80	70	65	55	50	45	40
40 Kg			90	80	75	65	55	50	45
44 Kg		120	100	85	80	70	60	55	50
48 Kg	165	130	110	95	85	80	65	60	55
53 Kg	180	140	120	105	95	85	75	65	60
58 Kg	190	150	130	115	105	95	80	70	60
63 Kg	205	160	140	120	110	95	85	75	65
69 Kg	215	170	150	130	115	100	90	80	70
75 Kg	225	180	155	135	120	110	95	85	70
75+ Kg	235	190	160	140	125	115	100	85	75

Table 6.2 Female Weightlifting Classification

The Athlete's Perspective

Weightlifters benefit from this system because they can compare their performances between classes. It provides them with clear goals. They can judge their successes by how quickly they move up through the classes. The more talented athletes will move quickly from Class 3 up to Master of Sport. The less talented ones may never get to Master of Sport. Less talented weightlifters might also struggle just to move from Class 2 to 1.

This will provide a perspective for the athlete on how well suited or talented he or she might be for the sport. This perspective can be used to ground an athlete who is too elated with his or her progress or relative success within his age group, or it can be used to provide the athlete with a measuring stick to determine the amount of progress that has taken place. In any case, it is one of the functions of the coach to use the Class system to keep the athlete focused on the training ahead.

For others, it just might supply the incentive needed to persevere and adapt to the training demands of the sport. I've always been an advocate of weightlifters training in a group setting as it allows for the establishment of culture. Class rankings can provide some of the benchmarks around which the group can develop values. They would become another means of comparison between athletes of both genders in different bodyweight classes.

The Coach's Perspective

The Classification System provides a great advantage for coaches wishing to determine the rate of progress of the weightlifters they are coaching. Instead of just using the improvement rate by kilos, which is going to vary depending upon gender, bodyweight and age, the coach can use the class rankings as an additional measuring stick. Whereas one athlete might make a 10 kg improvement that is significant, another may make a 15 kg improvement that is not as meaningful.

The coach can then compare how much closer an athlete is to the next class level. For instance if one athlete is 15% away from achieving a Class 1, then a 10 kg improvement may have a certain meaning, whereas the same increment might not be as meaningful to the lifter attempting to achieve a Class 2 ranking.

Furthermore, the Class ranking of a lifter will also determine the degree of rigor and the character of training to be planned to continue making progress along the PASM pathway. Although every athlete is somewhat unique, most coaches will find it most expeditious to group lifters by Class, and then secondarily by bodyweight class groups based on metabolic considerations.

Bodyweight class groups for men should be 56 and 62 kg in a first group, 69 and 77 in a second group, 85 and 94 in another and 105 and +105 in another. Women can be grouped in a 48, 53, 58 first group, a 63 and 69 in a second group, and a 75 and +75 in a third group.

Terminology

As in all disciplines, some standard terminology must be agreed upon in order to make sure all coaches, researchers and athletes are dealing with the same concepts. Some of these terms are part of the American sports training lexicon, but they are not standardized to the degree of specificity needed to communicate accurately. Several of the terms have specific mathematical definitions that must be adhered to in order to accurately define the quantitative aspects of training.

A Brief Weightlifting Training Lexicon

Volume: The number of repetitions performed with weights in the intensity range from 60% to 105% assigned or attempted for an exercise, a training session, a microcycle, a mesocycle, or a macrocycle.

Repetitions Per Set: The number of repetitions performed in a set, before resting briefly and attempting another set (unless it is the final set of an exercise). This is a critical parameter, the importance of which is often not apparent to some coaches.

Intensity: The number of kilograms lifted per repetition, or the percentage of maximum lifted per repetition.

Average Absolute Intensity: The average weight lifted per repetition expressed in kilograms. This parameter will prove to be of great importance in the calculation of the K-value.

Average Relative Intensity: The average weight lifted per repetition expressed as a percentage of the maximum. The maximum may be the heaviest weight lifted at the conclusion of the previous macrocycle, or the planned maximum for the conclusion of the current cycle. This figure is expressed as a percentage. This index has a greater value in evaluating some characteristics of training since it can represent a variety of exercises with different maxima and represent them on a common scale.

Average Absolute & Relative Intensity Example: If an athlete plans a 100% snatch of 130 kg and performs the training sequence 60%/3, 70%/3, (80%/3)3, the calculations for these figures are as follows:

Average absolute intensity: [3(.6x130) + 3(.7x130) + 9(.8x130)] / 15 = 96.2 kg

Average relative intensity: [(3 x.6) + (3x.7) + (9x.8)] / 15 x 100 = 74%

Load: The total amount of weight lifted per session, day, microcycle, mesocycle, macrocycle or year. This figure is calculated by multiplying the weight used in each set by the number of repetitions, and then adding all of these products to achieve a sum for whichever training unit is under consideration. This sum will be divided by the volume for the same training unit to achieve the average absolute intensity.

K-Value: This parameter is calculated by dividing the average absolute intensity by the total achieved at the concluding competition of the macrocycle, and then multiplying that quotient by 100. This is an index figure by which to determine the appropriate intensity of the training plan. *K-Value = (Average Absolute Intensity / Total) x 100*

Microcycle: A week's training.

Mesocycle: A training "month". This may be range in duration from 3 weeks (microcycles) to 5 weeks depending upon the class of the weightlifter.

Macrocycle: A long-term training program composed of 2 to 4 mesocycles organized in a periodized manner to achieve an optimal result in the concluding competition.

Periodization: The organization of long term training in such a manner that the body is subjected to an overreaching phase (preparation phase) followed by a restorative phase (pre-competition phase) that will result in supercompensation of the organism.

Preparation Phase: A period of 1 to 3 mesocycles characterized by larger training loads, medium-heavy average intensities and higher repetitions per set. Restoration is of extreme importance during this phase.

Pre-competition Phase: A period of 1 or 2 mesocycles during which the load is reduced and the average intensity is increased. The body is restored to a supercompensation state as the endocrines are restored and the nervous system is more highly stimulated.

Transitional Phase: A period of 1 to 3 microcycles that follow a pre-competition phase. They allow for restoration of the body before beginning on the next major macrocycle.

Concepts

The concept that must be primarily understood is that of supercompensation, the adaptation of tissue to a state of higher functioning through the inducement of stress. Other concepts that are supportive of supercompensation must also be understood, comprehended, assimilated and applied in order to fully implement a training program that leads to supercompensation.

Supercompensation is the result of a long-range program and is manifested in the competitive result at the end of the completion of a long-term training program.

The concept of training parameters as eu-stressors must also be mastered and manipulated. Their ability to impact the endocrine secretion is an important concept that must provide an overarching vision for the coach. The coach needs to understand when to raise the training load and when to raise the average training intensities in order to achieve the optimal results.

The concept of restoration of the organism after training sessions to increase the ability of the weightlifter to train with greater loads more frequently must also be understood and implemented if the training program is to be effectively conducted.

Finally, the concepts of muscular and connective tissue stimulation versus endocrine and nervous system disruption must be understood in order to manipulate the training parameters to achieve a harmonious result of the organism in the final competition.

Macrocycle

The macrocycle is basically the unit of planning. It is an extended period of time that runs from one meaningful competition to the next. It becomes more and more significant in the development of a weightlifter as the PASM reaches its advanced stages.

A macrocycle typically lasts from two to four "months" or mesocycles. The mesocycles are grouped as part of preparation phases or pre-competition phases. Typically a macrocycle is made up of a preparation phase and a pre-competition phase.

During the preparation phase(s) the training volume is large, though varied. The average absolute and relative intensities are medium-high. The variety of exercises is greater and the athlete is subjected to a condition of overreaching. The endocrines become fatigued and it is not uncommon for athletes to catch colds during the later portions of the preparation phases.

There is generally only one pre-competition phase. During this phase the training volume is reduced, the average absolute and relative intensities are raised. The variety of exercises is reduced and more classical lifts are performed and at higher intensities. The endocrines recover, and the nervous system is functioning at its optimal level during the final week.

Mesocycle

The mesocycle is a sub-unit of the macrocycle and might be referred to as a "month". Because it can vary in length from 3 to 5 weeks, it does not always conform to a calendar month. Generally the more advanced and heavier athletes will require longer mesocycles, while younger and lighter lifters will function best in shorter mesocycles.

During the course of a preparation mesocycle, there are loading (heavy) weeks, maintenance weeks and unloading weeks, whereas most of a pre-competition mesocycle is steady and gradual downloading.

Preparation Mesocycle

In a preparation mesocycle there are heavy, medium, and light "weeks" or microcycles. Since the average training week within a mesocycle does not vary significantly, the designation of heavy, medium or light refers to the variation in repetitions or volume. The mesocycle is assembled in such a way that the greatest amount of loading can be imposed while taking into consideration the relative placement of the given mesocycle within the macrocycle. A mesocycle might be made up of a sequence of microcycles designated as heavy-medium-heavy-light based on the volume. The next mesocycle might be heavy-heavy-medium-light with the greatest loading taking place at the end of the third microcycle.

Pre-Competition Mesocycle

In the pre-competition mesocycle, the microcycles might be organized in the sequence heavy-medium-light-very light, again based on volume. The average intensity will be significantly increased and the number of 90% intensity lifts will also increase during the pre-competition mesocycle.

During this period, the endocrines will restore themselves to supercompensatory levels, the muscles will be restored and the nervous system will achieve new levels of excitability.

Microcycle

The microcycle is a week of 7 days. Even if there is no training on a given day, it is still considered a part of the day count so that the effect on the organism can be maintained. Many training program microcycles have 6 training days with 1 rest day on Sunday. The Sunday rest day is considered a part of the training week so that training for the next microcycle does not begin on Sunday.

The microcycle during a pre-competition period may have two rest days for veteran lifters, and as many as three days for Class 2 and Class 3 lifters. These days must be maintained as rest days otherwise lifters may train too frequently or have too great a gap between training days in one week and the training days in the following week. Thus within the planning of a microcycle, the specific days of rest must be designated and considered an important part of the regimen both in number and sequence.

The Function of the Training Program at A General Level

The coach is the one who determines, in conjunction with the class ranking system, the correct level of the athlete and the appropriate training pathway. This pathway must be composed in such a manner that the athlete will achieve the greatest result during the prime competitive years. The training program must invoke the proper exercises in the proper sequences and in the proper dosages to ensure that the development is harmonious and convergent toward the prime athletic period.

The variables must be sufficiently implemented within reasonable ranges to ensure that the body is stimulated to generate the functional changes in structure and biochemical activity to lead to the most effective development. Concurrently, the psyche of the athlete toward the training and competitive processes must be developed through the organization of the training and competitive calendar.

In short, the coach must be keenly aware of the developmental processes in play and how they will be affected by the design of the training program. This is an educational and growth process for the coach.

CHAPTER 7
THE ROLE OF THE COACH

The coach is the organizer and the actual and cultural leader of a weightlifting program. Weightlifting is best developed in a group setting, as the training is so demanding that it is difficult to maintain the psychic energy to perform it without the company of other athletes. I've also found that a group of athletes do a better job of teaching, transmitting and reinforcing cultural norms to new athletes than I could ever do as a coach.

With respect to training, the coach designs the training and must be present to oversee the workout sessions. For this reason I do not advocate train-you-by-mail practices as I need to see the athlete on a daily basis as he or she proceeds through the training cycles. Whenever I have provided training programs for athletes I will not see regularly, I've felt compelled to let them know that they will have to make appropriate modifications on their own. This, of course, is not ideal. The coach should have some idea of what to expect at each stage of the macrocycle, and needs to know if the process is or is not unfolding as planned. Any unexpected trends of deviation must be detected fair quickly and addressed by modifications in the training plans.

During this process the coach should acquire a sense of what is normal for each athlete at each particular stage of the program. This regular observation is of great importance to the coach on the day of competition. During the weeks of the last mesocycle, the coach should pre-conceptualize a vision of the performance of the athlete. With this vision in mind, the coach can make appropriate physical and psychological adjustments during the course of the warm-up and competition.

Program Design

After a coach has been training weightlifters for several years, the process of program design should become one of second nature. In fact it is easy to develop a collection of boilerplate programs that are appropriate for each class level. Several times through a training cycle should provide a coach with the understanding to make appropriate modifications, especially to accommodate individual physical idiosyncrasies.

My approach is to have my lifters train in a group on the same basic program. I make individual modifications to deal with issues such as previous injuries, inherent weaknesses in structure or athleticism, bodyweight class, training age or age. Other factors that may enter into consideration are motor control inconsistencies, and local fatigue issues.

The training programs for the year should be laid out with respect to the events on the annual weightlifting calendar. These should be done with an eye to the meaningful competitions. These are national or international events depending upon the potentials of the individual athletes. For these competitions, the macrocycle is written with appropriate mesocycles designed to ensure a peak performance.

Local competitions that are for developmental purposes should be regarded as part of the normal training load for that week. There should be no cycling or downloading prior to those meets. In fact, I might even schedule an additional training session immediately after the competition. They can be helpful in terms of monitoring the progress of training at that point.

The number of macrocycles and their programming will also have to be modified for certain individual situations. If a junior lifter, for instance, is exceptional and is capable of qualifying for both the national junior championships and the national championships, there may not be time for a full macrocycle between the two events. A decision must be made as to the relative importance for each event.

The lifter in question may have a chance of winning the national juniors, qualifying for the junior world team, but has a lesser chance of placing highly at the national championships. In this situation the most important events are the juniors and the junior world's. The macrocycles must be programmed to peak for these events with specific peaking being designed for the nationals.

A truly exceptional junior might be so superior to the rest of the competition that a peak may not be necessary to win the juniors and qualify for the junior world team. In this case, the macrocycles must be planned to achieve the top peak at the junior world championships. In fact, we are seeking out this type of individual.

All of these types of decisions must be made as early as possible, although an unexpected result might bring up reason for further alterations. As an example, the macrocycle might be designed for a peak for the nationals and work effectively to the point where the lifter also qualifies for the continental championships. This will bring about a need to redesign the annual macrocycles.

One overriding consideration for program design is the annual volume. If the long-term goal is to achieve the greatest results possible, then the yearly plan must be adhered to in such a manner that the annual volume is not severely compromised. If 15,000 reps is the designated target volume, consistently altering the training by reducing the volume for insignificant competitions will inhibit the overall progress of the lifter.

It is tempting, especially early in the career of the coach, to become distracted by the relative success of the athlete in every major and minor competition. This is especially true if there is a parent who is swept up in the rapid progress of a talented young athlete and decides to intrude himself or herself in the training process. Part of the task of coaching is to take control of the situation and make decisions designed to advance the athlete along a pathway that will have the greatest long-term success.

One function of the program design is to establish goals for each meaningful competition. The goals should also include back squat and front squat performed during pre-designated training sessions. I prefer to use the goal weights as the means of calculating the percentages used in the training. The reason for this is that they keep the athlete psychologically focused on the goal weights so that by the time the competition arrives, the athlete has already visualized the lifting of these weights many times leading up to the meet.

Program Monitoring

There are two broad categories by which a coach can determine the effectiveness of the training program. The first is the daily observation of training. Although the absolute weights lifted could be reported back to a coach in absentia, this will in no way substitute for actually witnessing the training.

The reason for this is that the coach must be very attuned to the speed of the movements to determine the effectiveness of the training. For example, the third rep of a set at 80% will have a certain speed during the 4th week of a 12-week cycle, and perhaps a slightly different speed at the 10th week of that same macrocycle. The coach must be able to determine if the weight is moving at the appropriate speed (and it is an individual factor). If the weight is being lifted, but the speed is not consistent with the stage of programming, the training may have to be altered. The speed of the barbell and the speed of the athlete are key factors by which the coach can determine the effectiveness of the training. The more talented the athlete, the less variation there will be in speed of movement, and thus the task is doubly daunting when working with these lifters.

At certain points during the preparation mesocycles, the training may have to be somewhat curtailed on a particular day, or more reps may need to be added. These determinations can only be accurately made through direct observation.

I have used two indicators that allow me to realize that the training program is impacting the physiology of the athletes to an appropriate level. The first is the complaint of regular diarrhea. This usually occurs toward the end of the third week of a preparation mesocycle. The second indicator is when the athlete is waking up and falling back to sleep several times during the night. These are excellent indicators of overtraining or overreaching. My experienced athletes usually inform me when this is taking place, and I know they should be in this condition for about another week. The training may then have to be modified to allow for restoration of the organism.

Furthermore, specific occurrences in the non-weightlifting life of the athlete may bring about a disruption that will necessitate an alteration of the planned training. Although it is necessary for a coach to maintain a certain psychological distance from the athletes being coached, the lines of communication between coach and athlete should remain open in order for the coach to keep abreast of these types of non-weightlifting occurrences. These and other issues justify the presence of the coach at every training session.

At this point, I must interject a misconception about the role of a coach that is altogether too prevalent for many people outside of the sports world. A coach is not by intent a role model or a surrogate parent. The prime directive of the coach is to develop the athlete to the best possible outcome within reasonable means. A coach should be expected to fulfill this task in a most professional manner. While some coaches do periodically fulfill the role of a role model or surrogate parent, that is not their primary function, and both parents and athletes should not approach the training situation with those roles as preconceptions.

While sports are frequently viewed as a means for uplifting less fortunate youth, they should be first approached as an activity that has as its goal the development of athletic ability and the capacity to display that ability on demand. The primary criteria in determining the proficiency of a coach is the amount of knowledge and experience that is brought to the sport. Other aspects of the coach's individuality should be regarded as secondary considerations.

The K-Value

The K-Value is a derived figure that is calculated by dividing the total achieved at the end of a macrocycle into the average absolute intensity of the macrocycle. For the purposes of this calculation, closely missed lifts in training are included in the load, but very poor attempts or discarded reps (due to injury or excessive fatigue) are eliminated.

As an example, if an athlete has a result of 120 snatch and 150 clean & jerk at the end of a macrocycle for a total of 270, the K-value can be calculated by dividing the average absolute intensity into 270. If the athlete had a training load of 805,538 kg over the 20 weeks of the macrocycle and a volume of 7,653 reps, the average absolute intensity is 105.25 kg. 105.25 kg divided by 270 and multiplied by 100 yields a figure of 38.8. If this athlete has been training for several years, the K-value should then become a constant figure in the planning of training programs.

The meaningful range for Soviet athletes during the 1980's was from 38 to 42. For Bulgarians it was closer to 49.

I understand that the K-value of the most successful macrocycle is used as an index for writing future macrocycle plans by many successful coaches.

As the athlete reaches a higher classification level such as Class 1 or Candidate for Master of Sport, he or she is still in the process of determining the optimal K-value. The coach must take this into consideration when writing future training plans.

Competition Results

Meaningful competition results should have a great influence on determining the effectiveness of a given macrocycle program planning, and provide some possible directions for the designing of future training. After each such competition, the coach needs to evaluate the outcome in terms of a number of factors.

The success rate, the reason for failed lifts, the weight selection, the ability of the athlete to deal with the psychological aspects of competition, the effects of weight loss, weak areas in the body and the causes thereof, and any other relevant factors need to be taken under consideration in the designing of the next macrocycle.

Continued difficulty in making weight, relatively poor performances in the clean & jerk, and a general lack of improvement in the total of a developing athlete are also good indicators that the athlete needs to gain bodyweight and go up a class. This of course will necessitate a modification in the structure of training as bodyweight increases are a significant cause of alteration in the functioning of the body.

Above all, the coach needs to be evaluating the development of the athletes on the basis of performance, the development of training work habits and platform aplomb.

CHAPTER 8
DETAIL PLANNING

Once the coach understands the concepts of the PASM, GAS, homeostasis and periodization through either personal experience, and/or observing the training process under the tutelage of a master coach, the planning of training programs can commence. By the time that a coach is beginning this process, he or she should have some considerable experience with the sport. This acquaintance should allow the coach to accurately diagnose the relative strengths and weaknesses of the athlete in order that these factors can be considered in the program design.

The basic philosophy involved in the program design of a beginning level athlete is to plan training in such a manner that the athlete's development will become balanced with respect to the performance of the snatch and clean & jerk. For this reason a certain portion of the training must be given over to the remediation of weak areas. Weak areas in this context may not refer specifically to particular areas of the anatomy, but may also refer to motive qualities and physiological qualities.

Too many coaches with a background in some phases of weight training or physical therapy are too consumed with remediation of specific body parts, and not enough with training motive qualities and kinesthetic aspects.

Exercises

As the athlete undergoes the PASM, the number of exercises will diminish until the number is relatively small by the time that Master of Sport classification is achieved. During the early developmental stages of athletes (Class III and below), the number of exercises is large in order to remediate the weak aspects of the physical and motor development.

The coach needs to have a familiarity with the many available exercises and understand how to apply them and in what dosages, and most importantly when to discontinue them. Some body parts can be appropriately strengthened through correct performance of the classic lifts, but others will need specific remediation in the form of bodybuilding exercises or assistance lifts.

Besides strengthening specific portions of the anatomy, beginners may be in need of exercises to teach the proper usage of the legs in an explosive manner. Others may have difficulty conceptualizing the lowering of the body to place it under a barbell. Still others may be in need of special training to deal with a limited range of motion. Many newcomers may be in need of developing more local circulation through isolated body part training. All of these types of situations must be accurately diagnosed and the proper exercises prescribed in the appropriate dosages. This will be an ongoing process until the athlete reaches a relatively balanced state.

Another consideration is the development of training condition. This refers to the ability of the weightlifter to continuously undertake higher training loads for consecutive days. Some athletes that enter the sport late in life (early to mid-20s), may have the motive qualities, the proper range of motion and even the psychological skills, but because of the late start they are lacking in the capacity to regularly restore after demanding training loads.

Another factor to be considered is the psychological development of the athlete, and this aspect can be addressed through certain components of the program design, one of them being exercise selection and placement order within the training session.

All of these factors must be considered when the exercises are selected and in what volume they are prescribed to ensure that the training is rational in its approach to the development of the weightlifter.

Exercise Categories

Exercises are divided into categories to help with the exercise selection process. Each school of thought has its own grouping procedure. These groupings are structured to aid the coach in designing a well-rounded training program that ensures that the development of the lifter is balanced and functional with respect to competition.

Some of the groupings are done according to body part, while others are done according to phase of the movement. All of the grouping procedures are done in a rational manner. Coaches can then select an exercise from each grouping depending upon the state of development and the areas in need of remediation. The Romanians like to group their exercises into two broad categories, technique and strength. They have produced some great lifters so there is obvious merit to this system of designation as well. They and the Hungarians have also devised a system whereby each exercise is numbered according to its function. For instance all the snatch and snatch related exercises are in the 100 series, while all the clean & jerk exercises are in the 200 series. This means that coaches are writing programs with numbers representing the exercises to eliminate confusion.

The following grouping of exercises is provided as an example of how exercises can be grouped so that exercise selection is more effective and comprehensive. It is the result of studies conducted by former Soviet national coach, Alexei Medvedyev. They are taken from the text *A System of Multi-Year Training in Weightlifting* that was one of the study materials used at the Sport Institutes in the Soviet Union.

Medvedyev has divided the exercises into 9 groups according to their effect on the training, and the specific aspect or body part involved.

Fundamental Exercises (F.E.)

Snatch Exercises

Group 1:
1) Classic Snatch (The Squat Snatch)

Group 2:
2) Classic Snatch Below Knee Height: The lift commences with the bar being held off the floor, below the knee.
3) Classic Snatch at Knee Height: The lift commences with the bar held off the floor at knee height.
4) Classic Snatch Above the Knee: The lift commences with the bar held off the floor above knee height
5) Classic Snatch, Legs Straight: The lift commences with the legs straight
6) Classic Snatch Standing Straight: The lift commences with the bar held off the floor while the athlete is standing erect.
7) Classic Snatch on blocks: The lifter is standing on a block to begin the lift.

Group 3
8) Power Snatch
9) Power Snatch Below Knee
10) Power Snatch at Knee Height
11) Power Snatch Above Knee
12) Power Snatch, Legs Straight
13) Power Snatch on blocks
14) Power Snatch & Overhead Squat

Group 4*
15) Snatch Pull
16) Snatch Pull From Below Knee
17) Snatch Pull at Knee Height
18) Snatch Pull From Above Knee
19) Snatch Pull To Knee (Deadlift)
20) Snatch Pull on Block
21) Snatch Pull To Straight Legs: Snatch Pull until the Legs are straight, torso inclined forward.
22) Snatch Pull slow + Fast: Snatch Pull Slowly Plus a Fast Snatch Pull
23) Snatch Pull to Knee + Snatch Pull:

---

* There is no indication whether these are performed with a bending of the arms at the top of the movement or not. This issue is still a matter of debate among some coaches. In the programs that I write, I designate the pull with the arms bending as a high pull, and the pull with no arm pulling as an extension. I've found that both pulls have a place in the training. The Bulgarian training system that has been generally publicized does not indicate that pulls of any type are incorporated in the training of their elite athletes. This, however, is not a reason to believe that they have no place in the design of modern training methods.

24) Snatch Pull + Slow Down: Snatch Pull and then slow eccentric lowering
25) Snatch Pull + Below Knee + Above Knee: Snatch Pull, Snatch Pull below Knee, Snatch Pull above Knee
26) Snatch Pull 4 Stop: Snatch Pull with 4 3-second stops (at the instant of separation, at the knees, above the knees, and at heels raised)
27) Snatch Pull 4 Stop + Slow Down + Snatch Pull
28) Snatch Pull + Classic Snatch

Clean & Jerk Exercises

Group 5

29) Classic Clean & Jerk

Group 6

30) Classic Clean & Jerk Below Knee
31) Classic Clean & Jerk at Knee Height
32) Classic Clean & Jerk Above Knee

Group 7

33) Power Clean
34) Power Clean Below Knee
35) Power Clean at Knee Height
36) Power Clean Above Knee
37) Power Clean & Front Squat & Jerk
38) Power Clean & Power Jerk & Overhead Squat
39) Power Clean & Power Jerk

Group 8

40) Power Jerk off Rack
41) Power Jerk & Jerk off rack
42) Clean Grip Power Jerk & Overhead Squat
43) Half Jerk & Jerk: (I presume the Half Jerk is a Jerk Drive)
44) Jerk off Rack
45) Behind the Neck Jerk off Rack
46) Back Squat & Behind the Neck Jerk
47) Front Squat & Jerk

Group 9

48) Clean Pull
49) Clean Pull Below Knee
50) Clean Pull at Knee Height
51) Clean Pull Above Knee
52) Clean Pull to Knee (deadlift)
53) Clean Pull on Blocks
54) Clean Pull to Straight Legs

55) Clean Pull Slow & Clean Pull
56) Clean Pull & Slow Eccentric
57) Clean Pull Slow & Slow Eccentric
58) Clean Pull with 4 stops
59) Clean Pull with 4 stops & Clean Pull
60) Clean Pull with Medium Hand Spacing
61) Clean Pull to Knee & Clean Pull
62) Clean Pull and Clean

Squats

Group 10
63) Back Squat
64) Front Squat
65) Back Squat Slow Lowering & Fast Rise

Bend Overs

Group 11
66) Snatch grip Pulley Pull
67) Good Morning with Knees Flexed
68) Good Morning with Knees Flexed + Vertical Jump

Pressing

Group 12
69) Press
70) Push Press
71) Push Press & Overhead Squat
72) Behind the Neck Push Press and Overhead Squat
73) Snatch grip Behind the Neck Push Press and Overhead Squat
74) Pressing Snatch Balance
75) Bench Press (with clean width grip)

Exercises of Additional Loading (A.L.)

Exercises for the Legs

Group 13
76) Back Squat with Heels Raised
77) Leg Press on Leg Press Machine
78) Lunge, Barbell on shoulders
79) Lunge, Barbell on chest
80) Lunge, Barbell between legs
81) Vertical Jump Starting with barbell held below knees with snatch grip

82) Depth Jump

Exercises for the Back

Group 14
    83) Hyperextension
    84) Good Morning with Legs Straight
    85) Good Morning Seated on the Floor
    86) Good Morning Seated on a Bench

Exercises for the Arms and Shoulder Girdle

Group 15
    87) Snatch grip Behind the Neck Press
    88) Snatch grip Behind the Neck Press + Overhead Squat
    89) Squat Snatch Press
    90) Seated Press
    91) Incline Barbell Press
    92) Clean grip Straight Legged Snatch
    93) Snatch grip Straight Legged Snatch
    94) Clean grip Straight Legged Snatch & Overhead Squat
    95) Clean grip Straight Legged Snatch from Knee Height
    96) Thumbless Snatch Grip Straight Legged Snatch From Above Knee
    97) Clean grip Straight Legged Snatch from Above Knee
    98) Snatch grip Straight Legged Snatch from Above Knee
    99) Clean grip Straight Legged Snatch with legs and torso straight at start
    100) Snatch grip Straight Legged Snatch with legs and torso straight at start

Available Exercises

The preceding list of exercises is very exhaustive and for every situation that a coach might encounter in training, there is an appropriate exercise in the list. It is a very large menu, however. Since most workouts will normally not consist of more than 5 or 6 exercises, it is obvious that most of the 100 exercises will not be involved with any great regularity.

Some of the exercises are going to be used very frequently and they will make up the majority of the movements employed in a typical training program.

The list was developed during the period when training theory prescribed that the greater the variety of muscular stimuli, the greater the adaptation. Hence while only 23 exercises were recommended for the novice lifter, it was expected that by the time the athlete reached the Master of Sport level that all 100 exercises would be incorporated into the training.

Currently the long-term training plan incorporates the most exercises at the very beginning of training and the number dwindles down to a very small number for the elite level weightlifters.

At present a larger number of exercises are incorporated in the training of low level lifters in order to facilitate the learning of technique and to remediate the weak areas. Other exercises are added to ensure a synergistic development of the large muscle groups involved in the development of force, both from a muscular and neuromuscular perspective.

The choice of exercise is entirely dependent upon the developmental level of the athlete. While it is agreed that all lifters will have to perform some form of snatching, cleaning and jerking, and squatting in nearly all training sessions, the rest of the training exercises may be comprised of a large variety depending upon which areas are in greatest need of remediation.

Exercise Selection

Class 3 training sessions employ exercises in smaller numbers because of the lower volume. This precludes the inclusion of a range of exercises that stimulate the entire body in each workout. Most workouts feature one complete, explosive movement such as a classic snatch or a variant, a snatch derivative, a classic clean or a variant, or a clean derivative. A pulling or deadlifting exercise may follow that and then a squatting variant or additional leg strengthening exercise. The final exercise might be a remedial movement, which may or may not be counted in the volume.

Each of the snatch and clean variants should be included in at least 2 training sessions per week in order to reinforce the neuromotor patterns. Front or back squats should be included in at least two sessions per week (more if the athlete is in need of greater leg strength). Some type of pulling or deadlifting should be included in at least two workouts per week. Jerking or overhead strengthening movements should be included at least twice per week, again depending upon the individual strength of the individual.

The Class 3 weightlifter is young and physically immature, and therefore in need of strengthening movements in order to perform the lifts properly. Whereas some aspects of a snatch or clean may be relatively easy for a Class 3 athlete to perform, others may not be so easily performed. To balance out the development, supplemental exercises must be selected that will strengthen the weaker area. This must be a primary influencing factor in the selection of exercises beyond snatches, cleans, jerks and squats.

A Class 2 weightlifter is able to perform training sessions with both a classic snatch and a power clean in combination or a power snatch and classic clean & jerk combination. This is due to the way in which the training load (load, not volume) of the two exercises stresses the organism. Thus either of these two combinations may be scheduled for most training sessions. Depending upon other loading factors, these can then be followed with some type of pulling or deadlifting in most sessions. Back or front squats should be performed three times per week in most weeks with back squats outnumbering the front squats in a 2:1 ratio during the preparation phase. The ratio can be reversed during the pre-competition phase. The total number of remedial or supplemental strengthening exercises should be somewhat reduced from the Class 3 regimen.

Class 1 weightlifters should be fairly well balanced and approaching the proper bodyweight to height ratio. They may perform classic snatches and classic clean & jerks in the same workouts if the training load of the combination is compatible with the rest of the loading and volume. All training sessions should include supplemental pulling or deadlifting in sufficient variety. Full back and front squats should be performed three times per week in the same proportions as described for Class 2 lifters. The number of workouts per week will reach 5 in some preparation microcycles, and the distribution of exercises must be taken into consideration in order to ensure there is no excessive development of fatigue in a specific body part or region.

Candidate for Master of Sport and Master of Sport weightlifters will frequently have training sessions that include both classic lifts. Pulls or deadlifts are included in every session, and back or front squats may be performed six days per week during the heaviest preparation microcycles. The number of remedial or supplemental exercises is quite a bit smaller, and for some athletes may be almost non-existent.

International or Merited Master of Sport lifters will have the smallest number of exercises. The classic lifts may each be programmed for four of the six training days of the week, while power snatches and power cleans will be included in two of the training days. Back squatting and front squatting will be performed during each day of the heavier microcycles of the preparation mesocycles. Pulling movements will be performed in just about every session, save for the final week of the pre-competition. Pressing and some shoulder movements will be included quite frequently.

Repetitions Per Set Variation by Type of Exercise

Generally the number of repetitions per set will vary according to the category of exercise and the mesocycle. When programming the classic lifts and their derivatives, the number of repetitions per set should rarely exceed 4 and that only during certain days of the preparation mesocycles. On other days during those periods, the number can be less. The number should gradually diminish as the athlete enters the pre-competition mesocycle until the final two or three weeks prior to competition, when singles should predominate.

For squats, pulls, extensions and deadlifts, the number can be one or two repetitions higher, although following the same reduction pattern as the competition draws near.

For exercises designed purely for remediation, balancing or improving local circulation, the number can be as high as 10 or 12, and only be included for unclassified lifters.

Exercise Order

Once the exercises for a given microcycle (week) have been designated and divided into days, they must be placed in the correct order to have the greatest effect on the organism. The general prevailing principle is to use a speed and complexity of movement gradient to ensure that the speediest, most complicated movements are performed when the nervous system is at its freshest. At the early stages of development (Class 3), this may be deviated from periodically in order to address a particularly weak area in need of remediation.

For athletes that are in advanced stages of training (CMS, MS, IMS) it is acceptable to assign front or back squats to the beginning of the workout in order to pre-fatigue the legs before performing classic movements. This is done so that the nervous system will have to recruit less stimulated motor units to generate the contraction, thus training the nerves to stimulate more of the individual muscles' motor units.

This is especially effective for advanced lifters when the training day is broken up into multiple sessions. Less explosive movements are performed with the same effectiveness during morning trainings as they are in afternoon or evening sessions. Explosive movements are generally more effectively performed during the second session of the day.

The generally best sequence for assigning the exercises in a single workout is to select exercises from the various groups and order them so as to provide the athlete with a complete training of the major muscle groups involved in the performance of the snatch and clean & jerk. The first exercise should be the speediest, most complicated movement, and should provide primary stimulation for the pull.

This is obviously the snatch and/or the power snatch. These movements can be performed from the floor, from the hang or while standing on blocks. The clean & jerk is speedy, but less so than the snatch and so some variant of the clean & jerk and/or power jerk should be placed second.

During the class 2 and class 3 phases, specific leg work is generally scheduled for three sessions per week. The back squat or front squat should be included during these sessions with some attention being given to the specific weaknesses of the individual.

In the planning of training for Class 3 and perhaps Class 2 athletes, some workouts may be composed solely of slow, strengthening movements due to the fatigue level of the motor nerves, and the need for greater strength development in certain areas of the body.

The final portion of the training should be given over to exercises to strengthen areas in need of more stimulation or remediation. Pressing, rowing, hyperextensions and similar bodybuilding type movements are not especially taxing to the organism and will aid in the balancing of development. Those exercises listed as exercises of additional loading would fit into this category.

Percentages

Most of the world's training systems make use of percentages as a means of keeping track of the intensity of the training on a relative basis. So many training programs have traditionally prescribed a certain number of repetitions and a certain number of sets. Three sets of ten is a typically clichéd prescription, and although it works for certain purposes, the prescription lacks an intensity and is therefore not as effective as it could possibly be.

I've based all of the training programs I've written on four relevant maxima on which all the percentages are based. A small number of the exercises I've prescribed have optimal intensities that are not dependent on any of the four and they will be covered separately.

Some coaches prefer to use a 100% figure based on the best results achieved at the culminating competition at the conclusion of the last macrocycle. This is reasonable and workable and is especially more so as the progress of the athlete nears the end of the PASM and the increments of improvement are relatively small absolute figures. It, however, does not always focus the vision of the athlete forward. This is especially important for athletes during the early stages of development. I therefore select goal 100% weights at the beginning of each macrocycle.

Recently some systems have athletes max out each morning to determine 100% for the day. I have no definitive results to determine how effective this approach has been. In many cases, the coach may have to make alterations anyway as the training progresses, and this is where the judgment of the coach becomes of the greatest value.

The 100% Snatch: In the programs that I design, this is the goal weight for the end of the current macrocycle at the culminating competition. If the training is well designed, the athletes have come close to lifting this amount or may have actually lifted it during the final weeks of the pre-competition mesocycle, and are extremely confident of their abilities to lift the weight.

After training under a proper training system for a while, the athlete knows the meaning of a 90%, or a 95% single performed three weeks prior to a competition. He or she can judge by the speed and ease of the movement whether or not the 100% weight is a reality during the upcoming competition.

All snatch exercise intensities are based on this 100% figure. This includes snatch pulls, snatch deadlifts, snatch extensions, overhead squats and power snatches. For most athletes training under a well designed program scheme and with excellent technique, the 100% power snatch should fall in the 80—85% range of a 100% classic snatch. Some coaches write intensities for the power snatch based on a 100% figure for the power snatch, but I feel that it is a better integration of the benefits of the two movements if the same 100% figure is employed for both.

The range of percentages and the proportion of percentages is extremely important in the development of strength and speed-strength characteristics. 50% weights are generally not involved in the training of athletes from Class 2 on up.

Although a 50% weight (or weights of any percentage) can be somewhat inaccurate for an untried Class 3 lifter, weights of this intensity are helpful for learning proper motor patterns in some movements where heavier weights might prove to be unwieldy for a young, developing athlete.

Otherwise the prescribed intensities are in the 60% to 110% range. In general, the lower intensities will enhance speed qualities, while higher intensities will contribute more to strength increases. The intensity that most effectively and concurrently improves both speed and strength is 80%, provided that the technique of the athlete is well developed.

At this point a coach might wonder how one can perform lifts at intensity greater than 100%. The lifts that would employ 100%+ weights are pulls, deadlifts and periodically quarter or half squats, both front and back performed as remediation.

The 100% Clean & Jerk: This figure should be calculated to be in the range of 120% to 128% of the 100% snatch figure. This may not be realistic for Class 3 lifters, but it will become more feasible as the athlete advances through the classes. All clean exercises, clean extensions, clean high-pulls, clean deadlifts, Romanian deadlifts (initially), jerks, power jerks, push presses and any other clean & jerk related exercises should base their intensities on the 100% clean & jerk figure.

The 100% Back Squat: This figure should be at least 130% of the 100% clean & jerk target figure. Generally the higher the back squat figure, the lower the chance of knee injuries. All back squat exercise intensities, including ½ squats, ¼ squats, and eccentric squats, should be based on the 100% back squat figure.

The 100% Front Squat: This figure should be at the very least 105% of the 100% clean & jerk target weight. It would of course be valuable to have the front squat figure be higher, and this can hopefully be achieved as the development of the athlete progresses.

Some exercises do not have a consistent relationship to the four 100% figures defined earlier. For those exercises, usually pressing movements and good mornings, the weight selection will be within the purview of the coach.

Determining the Volume Within Percentage Zones

This is a difficult topic to comprehend easily as there are a number of different strategies that can be employed, and these may be modified depending on the individual circumstances. The coach will have to bear in mind the general principles at all times and make appropriate adjustments as they come about.

The intensities can generally be divided into 10% increments:

50—59%: Zone 1
60—69%: Zone 2
70—79%: Zone 3
80—89%: Zone 4
90—100%: Zone 5

There has been quite a bit of study to show that training excessively in high intensity zones will not aid in the development of speed, and that excessive repetitions performed in low intensity zones will improve speed, but impede the development of strength. Since both speed and strength are necessary components of weightlifting, intensities must be employed across a wide range. We also know that weights below 55% for Class 3 lifters and below 60% for Class 2 and above will have no effect on improving performance with respect to the development of speed and/or strength.

If we are using only the four maxima previously mentioned, then power snatches, power cleans and power jerks will provide most of the work in the zones that span 60%—75%. This will aid in the development of speed characteristics. Classic snatches, clean & jerks, back squats and front squats are spread out more evenly in the zones that span 60% to 100%, and in fact are similar to a normal distribution. Thus snatches and clean & jerks are responsible for developing both speed and strength characteristics. On the high end of the percentage scale, pulls, extensions, deadlifts, jerk drives, and partial squats will occupy the span of 80%—105%. Thus volumes will be assigned to each of the intensity zones.

If sufficient and appropriate volumes are assigned to each intensity zone, the average absolute intensity will yield a K-value within the prescribed 38 to 42 range. It is, however, obviously possible to have a bi-modal curve with much of the volume in the low and high zones and still calculate an average absolute intensity that leads to an appropriate K-value figure. So more specific planning must go into the designing of the training.

A number of studies have been done by the Soviets on high-level athletes and yielded the data, gathered by Medvedyev, presented in the following tables. These are not rules; they are simply the collected data. It is the job of the coach to properly interpret the data and apply those interpretations. Some knowledge of statistics and how to use the information in dealing with an athlete's physiology is a necessity. There are no results for Class 3 athletes as an accurate 100% figure is difficult to determine for a variety of reasons.

Table 8.1 details average relative intensity (ARI) and the number of 90 to 100% lifts performed in the snatch and clean & jerk exercises. Since the range is in the 90—100%, I believe we can presume that we are dealing solely with the classic lifts.

Qualification	Preparation		Pre-Competition		Transition	
	ARI	90—100%	ARI	90—100%	ARI	90—100%
Class 2	75.5	56	76.0	44	73.5	20
Class 1	75.0	44	76.0	56	76.0	32
CMS	72.5	20	74.0	28	72.5	12
MS	72.1	20	74.0	28	71.0	8
IMS	72.1	20	74.0	28	71.0	8

Table 8.1 Average Relative Intensity (ARI)

Table 8.2 presents data on the snatch for an annual period. The numbers in the zone columns are the percentage of all snatch repetitions performed in that zone. The ARI is the average percentage for the year, which may represent several different 100%s.

Qualification	Snatch Zones of Intensity					
	60—65%	70—75%	80—85%	90—95%	100%+	ARI
Class 2	9%	51%	29%	11%		75%
Class 1	7%	56%	28%	8%	1%	75%
CMS	10%	61%	25%	4%		72%
MS	16%	63%	19%	2%		71%
IMS	16%	63%	19%	2%		71%

Table 8.2 Zones of Intensity for the Snatch

Table 8.3 represents the one-year volume for the clean & jerk with the lifts represented as percentages of the total number and the ARI representing the average percentage.

Qualification	Clean & Jerk Zones of Intensity					
	60—65%	70—75%	80—59%	90—95%	100%+	ARI
Class 2	8%	42%	37%	12%	1%	76%
Class 1	4%	45%	39%	11%	1%	77%
CMS	9%	53%	33%	5%		74%
MS	11%	55%	31%		3%	73%
IMS	11%	55%	31%		3%	73%

Table 8.3 Zones of Intensity for the Clean & Jerk

Table 8.4 represents the same distribution for the snatch pull. As expected, there is a skewing toward the higher zones.

Qualification	Snatch Pull Zones of Intensity				
	80—85%	90—95%	100—105%	110%	ARI
Class 2	20%	41%	36%	3%	92%
Class 1	24%	33%	39%	4%	92%
CMS	31%	32%	31%	6%	91%
MS	25%	37%	32%	6%	91%
IMS	25%	37%	32%	6%	91%

Table 8.4 Zones of Intensity for Snatch Pulls

Table 8.5 provides the same distribution for the clean pull.

Qualification	Clean Pull Zones of Intensity					
	70—75%	80—85%	90—95%	100—105%	110%	ARI
Class 2	6%	30%	40%	20%	4%	89%
Class 1	17%	34%	26%	19%	4%	87%
CMS	23%	36%	23%	13%	5%	84%
MS	205%	38%	24%	13%	5%	84%
IMS	20%	38%	24%	13%	5%	84%

Table 8.5 Zones of Intensity for Clean Pulls

Table 8.6 provides the same distribution for squats. It is not specified as to whether they are back squats or front squats or both. I would guess that it is both.

Qualification	Squat Zones of Intensity					
	50—55%	60—65%	70—75%	80—85%	90—95%	ARI
Class 2	13%	28%	27%	30%	2%	71%
Class 1	14%	27%	21%	35%	3%	70%
CMS	22%	28%	25%	22%	3%	68%
MS	22%	30%	25%	20%	2%	66%
IMS	22%	30%	25%	20%	2%	66%

Table 8.6 Zones of Intensity for Squats

Table 8.7 takes into account the percentages of all the fundamental exercises with the exclusion of presses and good mornings. This may be the most helpful of all tables.

Qualification	Fundamental Lifts Zones of Intensity							
	50—55%	60—65%	70—75%	80—85%	90—95%	100—105%	110%	ARI
Class 2	3%	8%	28%	32%	16%	12%	1%	80%
Class 1	3%	11%	31%	31%	16%	7%	1%	78%
CMS	5%	11%	40%	26%	10%	6%	2%	79%
MS	4%	13%	39%	25%	10%	8%	1%	79%
IMS	4%	13%	39%	25%	10%	8%	1%	79%

Table 8.7 Zones of Intensity for Fundamental Lifts

Table 8.8 takes into account the percentages of all the exercises included in the sample 20-week program provided in this text. It is appropriate for a Master of Sport lifter and provides another set of figures that can be helpful in designing a training program.

Zone distribution for Master of Sport 20 Week Program					
% Zones	60—65%	70—75%	80—85%	90—95%	100%+	ARI
% of lifts	19%	24%	30%	11%	3%	76%

Table 8.8 Zones of Intensity for Master of Sport Program

Now while looking through all of this information, there are liable to be some contradictions. This is normal, as all of this information is empirical data and some of the generalizations are provided as guidelines, not as hard rules. Your capacity to make decisions based on empirical evidence is part of your toolkit as a coach.

Prilepin's Table

This table (Table 8.9) was developed by former Soviet national coach A.S. Prilepin in 1975 based on the training diaries of thousands of Soviet qualified (Class 1 and above) lifters. The numbers are specifically based on snatch and clean & jerk lifts and do not indicate how other fundamental exercise loading is varied. He studied two 5-week mesocycles and

Prilepin's Table		
Percent Zone	Rep Range/Set	Total Rep Range
70—75%	3 to 6	18
80—85%	2 to 4	15
90%	1 to 2	10 snatch / 7 clean & jerk

Table 8.9 Prilepin's Table

found that the best results were obtained in the first Mesocycle by lifting 90% weights and in the second by lifting 80% weights. This is another useful tool, among several, that can be used to plan an appropriate training program.

Progression Patterns

One of the skills that must be mastered by the coach is the pattern of intensity progressions, as well as progressions of repetitions per set.

Snatch and Clean progressions: A very simple progression that might be adequate for Class 3 lifters or for a second day or session of classical lifts might be 60%/2, 70%/2, 75%/2, 80%/2, in which the denominator is the number of repetitions in the set. For a workout to be effective, the intensity of the classic lifts must reach, at a minimum, 80%. The average intensity here is $[(60\% \times 2)+(70\% \times 2)+(75\% \times 2)+(80\% \times 2)]/8 = 71.25\%$

As the lifter improves from class to class, the emphasis on the intensities is to move toward more and more of the work being performed at 80%. Thus for a Class 2 lifter the previous progression might be changed to 60%/2, (70%/2)2, (80%/2)2. The calculation here would then be $[(60\% \times 2) + (70\% \times 4) + (80\% \times 4)]/10 = 72\%$.

For a Class 1 lifter, the progression would increase to 60%/2, 70%/2, (80%/2)3. The calculation of average relative intensity would then be $[(60\% \times 2) + (70\% \times 2) + (80\% \times 6)]/10 = 74\%$

For Candidate for Master of Sports (CMS), the progression would change to 60%/2, 70%/2, (80%/2)4. The calculation of average relative intensity would then be $[(60\% \times 2) + (70\% \times 2) + (80\% \times 8)]/12 = 75\%$

For Master of Sport (MS) and International Master of Sport (IMS), the progression changes to (80%/2)6. In this case the average relative intensity is 80%.

Two questions might arise here. One may wonder why do any sets with lower intensities if 80% has the greatest benefits for the increase of both strength and speed? The reason is that the lighter intensities (60%—75%) have an effect on the improvement of speed and the reinforcement of technique that is extremely important for the development of the developing lifter.

The second question that would come to mind is that if strength is more greatly affected by higher intensities, how does one incorporate heavier weights into the training. The intensities of 85%—100% will definitely increase strength, but they can also have a greater effect on the nervous system that will require more restoration. Of course some weights in these intensities ranges must be employed. Furthermore pulls with higher intensities are quite the norm.

In the sample programs found in each of the six chapters dealing with each specific class ranking, there are numerous examples of how the progressions are planned so as to incorporate all of these percentage range influences.

General Trends in Volume Over Class, Age, and Weight

Class: The general trend in volume is to gradually increase as one progresses from the beginning stage (7,000 reps per year) to Sports Mastery (25,000 reps per year).

Age: Provided that the athlete is beginning at an appropriate age (12—14), the volume will continue to rise until the age of approximately 27—30. At that point progress is still possible, but the athlete will have become more efficient and needs to reduce volume in order to avoid unnecessary injuries. This is the reason that volume figures are given as ranges.

Weight: On a very general level, the lighter the athlete, the greater the volume. At the Sports Mastery level (CMS and above), the 105 kg and +105 kg athletes will have the lowest volume on a consistent level. My personal experience with the larger lifters is that they are somewhat fragile and easily injured. Special vigilance must be attached to their training.

Summary

In the process of program planning, as in the process of writing or many other creative endeavor, the perfection is not in the planning but in the revision of the planning. Once a program is written, it must be implemented, observed, and finally individualized and revised. The artistry of coaching comes in determining which realm needs modification, and to what degree of modification is necessary.

SECTION D
PROGRAM PLANNING BY CLASS

The Process of Acquiring Sports Mastery (PASM) was previously discussed as a general principle. This section deals with the basic application of that principle in the training of the athlete. It may seem obvious to state that the training program must become progressively more demanding as the PASM continues, but to many just entering the sport and driven by ambition, it may seem appropriate to attempt the most demanding of training regimens without proper preparation. This approach will not achieve the optimal result.

Since the establishment of the Junior World Championships in 1975 and now the Youth World Championships and Youth Olympic Games, the age of competitive lifters has gradually gone down. The lifters that were in the past qualified as Class 3 were older than their modern counterparts. Whereas lifters formerly began training during the mid-teens, modern lifters are beginning training at the age of 12 or even younger in some cases.

Prior to the mid-1970s, conventional wisdom held that weightlifting was a sport for the mature athlete and most organized programs did not seriously consider training athletes younger than 18. Since that time a great deal of data has been accumulated to show that the best results are realized when athletes begin their preparation at a much younger age.

The training strategy must be approached along several fronts. Training must first begin as a very generalized approach designed to enhance the athleticism of the individual. The groundwork must be established for developing the various organs and systems that will support the organism during future training. The nervous system must also be developed so that certain functional neuromotor patterns will be established and strengthened. The motive qualities and athletic psyche must also be addressed.

During the initial phase of training (prior to achieving Class 3 results), a good portion of the work must be devoted to mastering the technique of the classic lifts. An athletically talented youngster should be able to learn the technique of the snatch and clean & jerk with relative ease. The lifts are not particularly challenging in their technicality when compared to the results expected of gymnasts and figure skaters of comparable age.

Other basic athletic skills should also be part of the developmental training of the pre-pubertal athlete. This is one part of the General Physical Preparation (GPP). Another aspect is the development of the lungs, heart and circulation. Sound cardiopulmonary development will aid in the restoration of the individual as the training becomes more demanding.

The playing of competitive sports must also be emphasized in order to develop the athlete's psyche and performance aplomb.

Thus the athlete entering the pubertal period should come in with a soundly developed functional technique for performing the snatch and clean & jerk, an enhanced development of the vegetative qualities of the organism and the capacity to perform well during competitive situations.

The Class 3 training should be composed of a moderate volume spread throughout the year, combined with more GPP. The weightlifting exercises should further refine the technique, balance the body for the performance of the classic lifts, and stimulate strength development. The GPP activities will be implemented to continue the development of the vegetative functions. Very talented athletes may achieve the Class 3 standards within a short period of time.

The Class 2 training should see a reduction in the GPP and an increase in the annual training volume. Whereas the number of strengthening exercises may have been quite large in the Class 3 training, they will be reduced as the body becomes more balanced for performing the classic lifts. There will be a greater emphasis on strengthening the body overall and increasing the capacity of the body to sustain greater training loads.

Class 1 training should be geared to a more mature athlete. There is little or no GPP, little remediation and more of the training load is given over to performing the classic lifts and strengthening exercises. Some attention is also directed toward further increasing training capacity. The trainings should become more frequent and restoration should be a part of the regimen.

Candidate for Master of Sport, Master of Sport and International Master of Sport are categories for the mature athlete who can devote himself or herself to semi-full or full-time training. This is because the daily regimen, including restoration activities, will occupy so much of the day that school or a job can be too draining and intrusive to maintain. The average intensity will gradually rise as will the load and volume. The variety of exercises will continue to become narrower. The preparation mesocycles will prove to be especially demanding on the body and require a well-managed restoration regimen.

CHAPTER 9
CLASS 3 TRAINING

Class 3 athletes, as a group, are in need of many influences if they are to embark on successful careers as weightlifters. Not only are they in need of the proper training and technical lessons, but they are often lacking in their capacities to pursue goals, and to live the type of life that will enable goals to be realized.

Thus one of the major tasks of a coach is to provide the athlete with experiences and situations that will make this an educational experience with respect to goal achieving. Many of them will like weightlifting, but may not be as passionate as a more advanced athlete. Too many of them will have friends that are not committed to any activities and those friends can prove to be rather distracting. It is consequently the task of the coach to begin the process of educating the weightlifter how to deal with such distractions and social influences.

Much of this can be taken care of if the coach has trained a group of weightlifters beforehand who can provide a psychic ambience in which the novice or Class 3 lifter can learn to function. This social proof of appropriate behavior will lessen the teaching load of the coach and allow the coach to spend more time on the actual coaching of the intricacies and necessities of the sport.

Male weightlifters who have achieved the totals in Table 9.1 are considered Class 3. Female weightlifters who have achieved the totals in Table 9.2 are considered Class 3.

Weight Class (kg)	32	34	38	42	46	50	56	62	69	77	85	94	105	+105
Total (kg)	60	65	70	80	90	105	120	130	145	160	170	175	185	190

Table 9.1 Class 3 Men Qualification

Weight Class (kg)	32	36	40	44	48	53	58	63	69	75	+75
Total (kg)	50	55	65	70	80	85	95	95	100	110	115

Table 9.2 Class 3 Women Qualification

The training is designed for beginning level weightlifters who are not only learning the correct performance of the lifts, but are also in the process of remolding the development of the body to accommodate the performance of the lifts and the loading of the training. Consequently a great many more repetitions are performed in what might be considered bodybuilding or remedial exercises simply to achieve the balanced development.

In the perfect model, athletes in this classification are between 12 and 17 years of age. Prospective talents should not spend more than 2 years in this classification, and most will achieve the levels of the next class in a year of training. For those athletes who are especially prodigious in their talent, they may need no more than 3 or 4 years to move from Class 3 to Candidate for Master of Sport.

Of course one of the factors is the ultimate height of the individual. Athletes who are short of stature with short parents will achieve maturity at a relatively young age (14 or 15) and as such are capable of beginning training that is normally geared toward adults. The normal prescription for volume may in fact have a negligible effect on the physiology of the organism.

Exercise Selection

The exercises to be employed for this group are many and varied as the development of the athlete is going from general fitness to specialized weightlifter. Because much of the early work is spent on the development of technique and the balancing of the development of the body to perform the snatch and clean & jerk, the parameters of loading may not be closely adhered to.

Of course the classic lifts must be included to a certain extent, but much of the work must be given over to basic strengthening with back squats, front squats, presses, lunges, good mornings and deadlifts. The power clean, power snatch and power jerk must also be used in some frequency in addition to specialized auxiliary exercises for the trunk. Much attention must be given to learning portions of the technique of the snatch and clean & jerk, both to develop technique and to strengthen the specific musculature through the specific range of motion.

The 30 Most Appropriate Exercises to be Included in the Training of a Class 3 lifter:

1) Snatch
2) Clean & Jerk
3) Clean
4) Jerk Off Rack
5) Hang Snatch (from off the floor, below the knee, above the knee)
6) Hang Clean (from off the floor, below the knee, above the knee)
7) Power Snatch
8) Power Clean
9) Power Jerk (Snatch and Clean grip, In front of and back of the Neck)
10) Snatch Pull (or Extension)
11) Clean Pull (or Extension)
12) Back Squat
13) Front Squat
14) Romanian Deadlift
15) Snatch Deadlift
16) Clean Deadlift
17) Overhead Squat

18) Good Morning
19) Presses (Jerk and Snatch Grips, In Front of and back of the Neck)
20) Push Press (Jerk and Snatch Grips, In Front of and Back of the Neck)
21) Bench Press
22) Seated Press
23) Squat Snatch Press
24) Jerk Balance
25) Jerk Recovery
26) Jerk Lockout
27) Jerk Support
28) Abdominal Work
29) Hyperextensions
30) Pull-ups

It is the function of the coach to select the exercises, as well as the frequency of inclusion and the volume within the program.

Many exercises are designed to strengthen specific body parts to balance them with the rest of the development so that they are not in jeopardy of being injured while performing relatively heavy lifts. This is a particular concern with the highly talented, exceptional motor learner who can master the technique of the lifts in a very short period of time.

My experience has been that athletes with backgrounds in dance, gymnastics, figure skating and diving find the Olympic lifts to be relatively easy events to master from a technical standpoint. As a result they are capable of lifting weights that can be excessively stressful on the connective structures if not the muscles. The training programming for these athletes has to be geared much more toward strengthening than that employed for less talented individuals.

Most of the workouts (66% to 75%) must include at least one and preferably two exercises that are either the classic lifts (snatch and clean & jerk) or derivatives (power snatch, power clean, power jerk, jerk off rack). At least half the sessions should include back squatting or front squatting. Much of the remainder of the session must be devoted to strengthening exercises such as pulls, presses, lunges and good mornings. A certain percentage of most workouts should include specific body part exercises that are devoted to the remediation of weak areas. Some of the training sessions may be entirely devoted to strengthening movements. The shorter sessions may be supplemented with GPP activities and/or competitive games.

Yearly Loading Parameters and Other Considerations

The ideal range of the annual volume for Class 3 athletes is from 7,000 to 9,000 lifts. The range of the number of these lifts that are snatches and clean & jerks in the 90 to 100% range is from 200 to 300 lifts. The average range of the relative intensity of snatches and clean & jerks should be 65% to 75%. The recommended number of meaningful competitions is 4 to 5. A recommended maximum number of hours for weightlifting training is 12 hours per week.

Graph 9.1 displays the number of repetitions performed each week by a Class 3

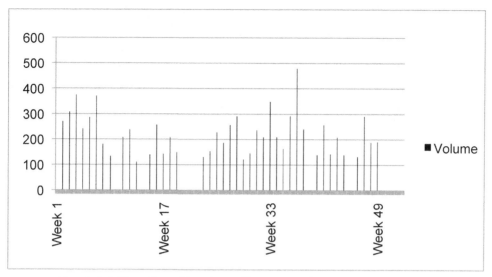

Graph 9.1 Class 3 weekly volume. The annual distribution of volume by weeks for a Class 3 lifter as proposed by Medvedyev.

lifter who is attending the Sport School. The bars provide an idea of how training is varied in a cyclical manner. The weeks with no vertical bars are competition weeks and the repetitions performed in those weeks are not counted as part of the yearly volume. Competitions are scheduled for Weeks 10, 14, 20, 39, 45, and 50. There are two-week breaks scheduled during the 21st, 22nd, 51st and 52nd weeks.

The figures provided in this section are not to be slavishly followed, but are here to provide some idea of how the volume is distributed, and to provide a representation of the concept of periodization.

Each week represents three to four workout days per week in most cases. These days are more or less evenly distributed, and during many of the interim days, the activity taking place is of a GPP nature.

During the weeks when no weightlifting training is scheduled, the lifter is participating in GPP activities that will continue to develop the vegetative qualities of the athlete for the training loads to be undertaken in the future.

Calculations

Annual Volume The process of program planning begins with the allocation of volume properly in the units of months (mesocycles), weeks (microcycles) and then days. This process is made all the more difficult by the fact that the athlete is still in a developmental state and may not respond as effectively as expected of a more experienced athlete. Nonetheless, the process must be attempted with the coach making appropriate adjustments as the procedure progresses.

The number of repetitions for the first year is prescribed at 7,000 to 9,000. I've found that the best results are obtained by planning one preparation month followed by a pre-competition month. The pre-competition month should be followed by a transition week. This adds up to a total of 9 weeks per macrocycle. The athlete can therefore plan on 5 9-week macrocycles or 45 weeks of the training year.

Four weeks may be given over to vacation. These vacation weeks should be interspersed throughout the year so that the athlete does not have a single four-week break. This accounts for 49 weeks of the year. The 3 additional weeks can be added to preparation mesocycles to increase the training volume.

Monthly Volume If 48 weeks are given over to training, this breaks up the year into 12 4-week mesocycles. For a total annual volume range of 7,000 to 9,000 reps, this breaks down to an average range of 583 to 750 reps per mesocycle. For a two-mesocycle period, this calculates out to a range of 1,166 to 1,500.

Since a reasonable ratio of preparation mesocycle volume to pre-competition volume is 1.5:1, it is possible to divide the aforementioned range by 5 for a quotient range of 233 to 300. Since the preparation month is made up of 3/5 of the time and the pre-competition month is 2/5, the range of reps is calculated as 699 to 900 for the preparation mesocycle and 466 to 600 for the pre-competition mesocycle.

Having calculated the ranges for the mesocycle or "month", the calculation of the weekly volumes can commence.

Weekly Volume In this volume range, the best distribution of volume for the four weeks is in the following percentages 35%, 28%, 22% and 15%. In an example of gradually descending weekly volumes, this means that 35% of the monthly volume is performed during week 1, 28% during week 2, 22% during week 3 and 15% during week 4. They do not have to be planned in this order, but the coach must keep in mind that the final week will impact the first week of the following month.

For the preparation month with a range of 699 to 900 reps, the weekly volumes will have the ranges shown in Table 9.3.

If the exercises and percentages are properly assigned, these ranges will find that 63% of the volume will be lifted in the first two weeks, causing an impact on the endocrines. The 3rd and 4th weeks will account for 37% of the reps. Some of this time in the third week will be given over to recovery from the first two weeks, but the very light volume of the fourth week will allow for a high volume in the first week of the following month.

Another effective distribution of the weekly volumes might be 35%, 22%, 28%, 15% or even 35%, 15%, 28%, 22%. These sequences can be adjusted by the coach as is

Week	1 (35%)	2 (28%)	3 (22%)	4 (15%)
Volume Range	245—315	196—252	154—198	105—135

Table 9.3 Class 3 Preparation Mesocycle Volume

Week	1 (35%)	2 (28%)	3 (22%)	4 (15%)
Volume Range	163—210	130—168	102—132	69—90

Table 9.4 Class 3 Pre-competition Mesocycle Weekly Volume

deemed necessary by the response of the athlete.

The arrangement of the weeks may be modified by the coach as necessary in response to the fitness of the athlete. It is generally beneficial to have the first week bear the largest volume. Many athletes, especially the younger and lighter ones, may still feel energetic at the end of the first week, and thus the second week can be of a sufficient load to further impact the body. The lightest week should be the last week as this provides for restoration before the next mesocycle commences.

For the pre-competition month with a range of 466 to 600 reps, the weekly volumes will have the ranges shown in Table 9.4. In a pre-competition month, the weekly volumes can also be rearranged, but Week 4 should always have the lowest volume since it immediately precedes the competition.

Daily Volume The weekly volume can now be distributed into the daily volumes with the following prescribed percentages. These percentages are being presented in ascending order. They are not necessarily to be assigned during these days. The training days are designated in Table 9.5 to show the distribution of training sessions throughout the week.

These daily volumes can also be arranged in different sequences while keeping in mind how the volume from a given day might impact the training in a subsequent session. A day of large volume should be followed by a day of light volume or rest in order to allow the body to take on a larger volume on the next training day.

For a Class 3 athlete, the optimal number of trainings is generally in the 3 to 4 per week range. During exceptionally high-volume weeks, a five-day training week may be planned. For a Class 3 athlete with a preparation mesocycle week of 300 reps, the volumes might be distributed over 4 training days as follows: Day 1: 105 (35%), Day 2: 45 (15%), Day 3/; rest, Day 4: 84 (28%), Day 5: 66 (22%), Day 6: rest, Day 7: rest.

Sample Training

With the following guidelines in place, and a list of available exercises available for selection the calculations can be made to determine the volumes for each training day.

For a macrocycle composed of one preparation mesocycle and one pre-competition mesocycle, the volumes can be represented in the Tables 9.6 and 9.7 and Graph 9.2. The percentages in the tables represent the repetitions or volumes, and not the intensity of

Workouts/Week	Day 1	Day 2	Day 3	Day 4	Day 5	Day 6
3	26%		32%		42%	
4	15%	22%		28%		35%
5	13%	15%	15%		27%	30%
6	11%	11%	11%	19%	22%	26%

Table 9.5 Class 3 Daily Volume

the weights.

From the repetitions represented in the daily volume columns, the specific training program can be derived as far as training volume is concerned.

Notation Conventions in the Standard Programs

The percentage figures provided are based on the four 100% maxima described in Chapter 8. The denominator is the number of repetitions performed with that intensity. If there are parentheses, the coefficient is the number of sets. For compound exercises, e.g. power snatch & overhead squat (60%/3+3), the first number of the denominator is the number of repetitions for the first exercise, and the second number is the number of

Preparation Mesocycle (900 reps)												
Weeks	1			2				3			4		
Weekly Percent	22%			35%				15%			28%		
Weekly Volume	198			315				135			252		
No. of Days	3			4				3			3		
Days	M	W	F	M	Tu	Th	Sa	M	W	F	M	W	F
Daily Percent	42%	26%	32%	22%	35%	15%	28%	42%	26%	32%	32%	26%	42%
Daily Volume	83	51	63	69	110	47	88	57	35	43	81	66	106

Table 9.6 Class 3 Preparation Mesocycle Figures

Pre-Competition Mesocycle (600 reps)												
Weeks	5			6				7			8		
Weekly Percent	28%			35%				22%			15%		
Weekly Volume	168			210				132			90		
No. of Days	3			4				3			3		
Days	M	W	F	M	Tu	Th	Sa	M	W	F	M	Tu	Th
Daily Percent	26%	42%	32%	35%	15%	28%	22%	42%	32%	26%	42%	32%	26%
Daily Volume	44	71	54	74	32	59	46	55	42	34	38	29	23

Table 9.7 Class 3 Pre-competition Mesocycle Figures

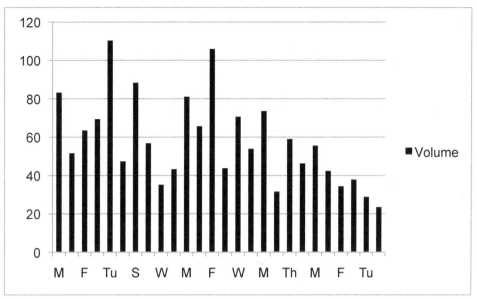

Graph 9.2 Class 3 daily volume. The graph of representing the daily volumes of a two-mesocycle macrocycle for a Class 3 weightlifter

repetitions for the second exercises. Whether the two exercises are performed in alternating pattern or if all the repetitions of the first exercise are completed before the second exercise is performed is left to the discretion of the coach. In the case of lunges, the two numbers represent the reps performed with the right leg forward and then the number of reps performed with the left leg, in no particular order.

The three numbers at the right of each line separated by colons represent respectively the number of repetitions performed in that particular exercise, the number of repetitions performed in that training day and the number of repetitions performed in that training week. Thus 12:52:135 means 12 repetitions of the given exercise are prescribed while 52 represents the number of repetitions performed that day and 135 represents the number of repetitions performed that week. This convention allows me to keep track of the training volume.

CL (12:52:135)
17 = CL in exercise
52 = CL in a day
135 = CL in that week

Prep Mesocycle = 900 Reps
Pre-comp Mesocycle = 600 Reps

SAMPLE CLASS 3 TRAINING PROGRAM

The numbers to the right represent respectively the number of repetitions in the exercise, the number of repetitions in the workout and the number of repetitions for the week.

Week 1 (Preparation Mesocycle) 198 repetitions   *22%.*

Day 1—Monday (83 repetitions) *42%*
1) Hang Power Snatch: 50%/3, 60%/3, 65%/3, (70%/2)2	13:13:13
2) Behind the Neck Power Jerk: 50%/3, 60%/3, (65%/3)2, (70%/2)2	16:29:29
3) Back Squat: 60%/3, (70%/3)2, 80%/3	12:41:41
4) Snatch Deadlift: (80%/3)2, (85%/3)2	12:53:53
5) Press: (X/4)4	16:69:69
6) Hyperextension: (X/7)2	14:83:83

Day 3—Wednesday (51 repetitions) *26%*
1) Clean: 50%/3, 60%/3, 70%/3, (75%/3)2	15:15:98
2) Front Squat: 60%/3, (70%/3)2, 80%/3	12:27:110
3) Push Press: 50%/3, 60%/3, 65%/3 (70%/2)2	13:40:123
4) Good Morning: (X/4)3	12:52:135

Day 5—Friday (63 repetitions) *32%*
1) Snatch: 50%/2, 60%/3, 70%/3, (75%/3)2, (80%/2)2	18:18:153
2) Back Squat: 60%/3, (70%/3)2, (80%/3)2	15:33:168
3) Clean Deadlift: (80%/4)4	16:49:184
4) Overhead Squat: 50%/3, (60%/3)2, (70%/3)2	15:64:199

Week 2 (Preparation Mesocycle) 315 repetitions   *35%.*

Day 8—Monday (69 repetitions) *22%*
1) Hang Power Clean: 50%/3, 60%/3, 65%/3, (70%/3)2	15:15:15
2) Snatch High Pull: 70%/3, (80%/3)3	12:27:27
3) Power Jerk: 60%/3, 65%/3, (70%/3)2	12:39:39
4) Bench Press: (X/4)4	16:55:55
5) Hyperextension: (X/7)2	14:69:69

Day 9—Tuesday (110 repetitions) *35%.*
1) Snatch off blocks: 50%/3, 60%/3, 65%/3, 70%/3, (75%/3)2	18:18::87
2) Power Clean: 50%/2, 60%/2, (70%/2)2	08:26:95
3) Jerk off Rack: 60%/3, 70%/3, (75%/3)3	15:41:110
4) Back Squat: 60%/4, (70%/4)2 (75%/4)2	20:61:130
5) Snatch Deadlift with 2 halts: (75%/3)2, (80%/3)3	15:76:145
6) Press: (X/4)4 16:92:161	
7) Good Morning: (X/6)318:110::179	

Day 11—Thursday (47 repetitions) *15%.*
1) Behind the Neck Push Press: 50%/3, 60%/3, 65%/3, (70%/3)2   15:15:194
2) Overhead Squat: 50%/4, 60%/3, 65%/3, 70%/3   13:28:207
3) Clean Deadlift: 70%/4, (80%/4)4   20:48:227

Day 13—Saturday (88 repetitions) *28%.*
1) Power Snatch: 50%/3, 60%/3, 65%/3, (70%/2)2   13:13:240
2) Clean & Jerk: 60%/3+2, 70%/3+2, 75%/2+1, (80%/2+1)2   19:32:259
3) Snatch High Pull: (80%/3)4   12:44:271
4) Front Squat: 60%/4, 70%/4, 75%/3, (80%/3)2   17:61:288
5) Lunge with bar between legs: (X/3+3)4   24:85:312

Week 3 (Preparation Mesocycle) 135 repetitions   *15%*

Day 15—Monday (57 repetitions) *42%.*
1) Snatch: 50%/2, 60%/2, 70%/2, 80%/2, 85%/1, 90%/1   10:10:10
2) Power Clean: 50%/2, 60%/2, 65%/2, (70%/2)2   10:20:20
3) Back Squat: 60%/3, 70%/3, 80%/3, 85%/2, 80%/3   14:34:34
4) Clean Deadlift: 80%/3, 85%/3, (90%/2)2   10:44:44
5) Press: (X/3)4   12:56:56

Day 17—Wednesday (35 repetitions) *26%.*
1) Overhead Squat: 50%/4, 60%/4, 65%/3, (70%/3)2   17:17:73
2) Front Squat: 60%/3, 70%/3, (80%/2)2, 75%/2   12:29:85
3) Good Morning: (X/3)309:38:94

Day 19—Friday (43 repetitions) *32%.*
1) Hang Clean: 60%/2, 70%/2, (80%/2)3   10:10:104
2) Jerk off Rack: 60%/2, 70%/2, (80%/2)2   08:18:112
3) Back Squat: 60%/2, 70%/2, 80%/2, (85%/2)2   10:28:122
4) Snatch Deadlift: 70%/3, (80%/3)3   12:40:134

Week 4 (Preparation Mesocycle) 252 repetitions   *28%*

Day 22—Monday (81 repetitions) *32%*
1) Clean & Jerk: 60%/2+1, 70%/2+1, 75%/2+1, (80%/2+1)2   15:15:15
2) Hang Power Snatch: 50%/3, 60%/3, 65%/3, (70%/2)2   13:28:15
3) Back Squat: 60%/4, 70%/4, (75%/4)2, (80%/3)2   22:50:50
4) Behind the Neck Push Press: 50%/3, 60%/3, 65%/3, (70%/2)2   13:63:63
5) Overhead Lunge: (X/3+3)3   18:81:81

Day 24—Wednesday (66 Repetitions) *26%.*
1) Snatch off blocks: 50%/3, 60%/3, 70%/3, 80%/3, 85%/1   13:13:94
2) Snatch High Pull off blocks: (90%/3)4   12:25:106
3) Front Squat: 60%/3, 70%/3, 80%/3, 85%/2, 75%/3   14:39:120
4) Power Jerk: 50%/3, 60%/3, 65%/3, 70%/3, 65%/2   14:53:134
5) Good Morning: (X/7)214:67:148

Day 26—Friday (106 repetitions) *42%*
1) Power Clean: 50%/3, 60%/3, 65%/3, 70%/3, 65%/3   15:15:163
2) Hang Power Snatch & Overhead Squat:
    50%/1+3, 60%/1+3, 65%/1+3, (70%/1+3)2   20:35:183
3) Clean Extension: 70%/4, (80%/3)3   13:48:196
4) Back Squat: 60%/3, 70%/3, (80%/3)2, (85%/2)2   16:64:212
5) Press: (X/4)4   16:80:228
6) Lunge: (X/3+3)4   24:104:252

Week 5 (Pre-competition Mesocycle) 168 repetitions *28%*

Day 29—Monday (44 repetitions) *26%*
1) Snatch: 60%/2, 70%/2, 80%/2, 85%/2, 90%/1   09:09:09
2) Power Clean & Power Jerk: 50%/3+3, 60%/2+2, 65%/2+2, 70%/2+2   18:27:27
3) Front Squat: 60%/3, 70%/3, 75%/3, 80%/3, 85%/2 80%/3   17:44:44

Day 31—Wednesday (71 repetitions) *42%*
1) Power Snatch & Overhead Squat:
    50%/3+3, 60%/2+2, 65%/2+2, 70%/2+2   18:18:62
2) Clean: 60%/2, 70%/2, 75%/2, 80%/2, 85%/2, 90%/1, 85%/2   13:31:75
3) Snatch High Pull: 80%/3, 85%/2, (80%/3)2   11:42:86
4) Back Squat: 60%/3, 70%/3, 80%/3, 85%/2, 80%/3   14:56:100
5) Press: (X/3)5   15:71:115

Day 33—Friday (54 repetitions) *32%*
1) Snatch High Pull & Snatch: 60%/2+2, 70%/2+1, 80%/2+1, 85%/2+1   12:12:127
2) Hang Power Clean: 50%/3, 60%/3, 65%/3, 70%/3   12:24:139
3) Front Squat: 60%/2, 70%/2, 80%/2, 85%/2, 80%/2   10:34:149
4) Clean High Pull: (80%/2)4   08:42:157
5) Bench Press: (X/3)4   12:54:169

Week 6 (Pre-competition Mesocycle) 210 repetitions *35%*

Day 36—Monday (74 repetitions) *35%*
1) Snatch: 60%/2, 70%/2, 80%/2, 85%/2, 90%/1, 85%/2   11:11:11
2) Power Clean & Power Jerk:
    50%/2+2, 60%/2+2, 65%/2+2, (70%/2+2)2   20:31:31
3) Snatch Deadlift with 2 halts: (80%/3)4   12:43:43
4) Back Squat: 60%/3, 70%/3, 80%/2, (85%/2)2, (90%/1)2   14:57:57
5) Push Press: 50%/3, 60%/3, 65%/3, (70%/3)3   18:75:75

Day 37—Tuesday (32 repetitions) *15%*
1) Clean & Jerk:
    60%/2+2, 70%/2+2, 80%/2+1, 85%/2+1, 90%/1+1, 85%/2+1   19:19:94
2) Clean Extension: (80%/3)4   12:32:106

Day 39—Thursday (59 repetitions) *287.*
1) Hang Power Snatch; 50%/3, 60%/3, 65%/2, (70%/2)3   14:14:120
2) Snatch High Pull: 80%/3, (85%/2)3   09:23:129
3) Front Squat: 60%/3, 70%/3, 80%/3, 85%/3, 90%/2, 85%/3   17:50:146
4) Press: (X/3)3   09:59:155

Day 41—Saturday (46 repetitions) *227.*
1) Power Clean: 50%/3, 60%/3, 65%/3, (70%/3)2   15:15:170
2) Jerk off rack: 60%/3, 70%/3, 75%/3, (80%/3)2   15:30:195
3) Clean deadlift: (85%/3)5   15:45:210

Week 7 (Pre-competition mesocycle) 132 repetitions *227*

Day 43—Monday (55 repetitions) *4/7.*
1) Snatch: 60%/1, 70%/1, 80%/1, 85%/1, 90%/1, 95%/1, 90%/1   08:08:08
2) Clean & Jerk: 60%/1+1, 70%/1+1, 80%/1+1,
       85%/1+1, 90%/1+1, 95%/1+1, 90%/1+1   16:24:24
3) Front Squat: 60%/2, 70%/2, 80%/2, 85%/2, 90%/1, 95%/1, 85%/2   12:36:36
4) Snatch High Pull: (85%/2)4   08:44:44
5) Press: (X/3)4   12:56:56

Day 45—Wednesday (42 repetitions) *327.*
1) Power Snatch: 50%/2, 60%/2, 65%/2, 70%/2, 75%/1   09:09:65
2) Power Clean & Power Jerk:
       50%/2+1, 60%/2+1, 65%/2+1, 70%/2+1, 75%/1+1   14:23:79
3) Clean High Pull: 80%/3, 85%/2, (90%/2)2   09:32:88
4) Back Squat: 60%/2, 70%/2, 80%/2, 85%/2, 90%/2, 95%/1, 85%/2   11:43:99

Day 47—Friday (34 repetitions) *267.*
1) Snatch: 60%/1, 70%/1, 80%/1, 85%/1, 90%/1, 95%/1   06:06:105
2) Clean & Jerk:
       60%/1+1, 70%/1+1, 80%/1+1, 85%/1+1, 90%/1+1, 95%/1+1 12:18:117
3) Front Squat: 60%/2, 70%/2, 80%/2, 85%/2, 90%/1, 95%/1, 85%/2   12:30:129

Week 8 (Pre-competition mesocycle) 90 Repetitions *154*

Day 50—Monday (38 repetitions) *427.*
1) Snatch: 60%/2, 70%/2, 80%/2, 85%/2   08:08:08
2) Clean & Jerk: 60%/2+1, 70%/2+1, 80%/2+1, 85%/2+1   12:20:20
3) Front Squat: 60%/2, 70%/2, 80%/2, 85%/2   08:28:28
4) Press: (X/3)4   12:40:40

Day 51—Tuesday (29 repetitions) *327.*
1) Power Snatch: 60%/2, 65%/2, (70%/2)2   08:08:48
2) Power Clean & Jerk: 60%/2+1, 65%/2+1, (70%/2+1)2   12:20:60
3) Back Squat: 60%/2, 70%/2, (80%/2)2   08:28:68

267.

Day 53—Thursday (23 repetitions)
1) Power Snatch: 60%/2, 65%/2, 70%/2   06:06:74
2) Power Clean & Jerk: 60%/2+1, 65%/2+1, 70%/2+1   09:15:83
3) Snatch: Extension: (80%/2)4   08:23:91

Day 55—Saturday
Competition

At this competition the athlete should be capable of lifting personal records in the snatch and clean & jerk provided that the psychological preparation has been appropriate and that the warm-up is well managed and the competition weights have been properly selected.

After the competition, the task of the coach is to determine whether or not the training was effective, to what extent it was effective and what modifications need to be administered in the next macrocycle.

CHAPTER 10
CLASS 2 TRAINING

Class 2 training is much more in line with classic program planning since the exercise selection is somewhat more limited. The technique of the lifts has been well ingrained into the motor patterns of the athletes, and the training can be planned with an eye toward two major goals: 1) the improvement of performance, and 2) the capacity to deal with greater training loads in future years. Secondarily the continuing education of the athlete in terms of competitive prowess and adapting the lifestyle is ongoing.

Male weightlifters who have achieved the totals in Table 10.1 are considered Class 2. Female weightlifters who have achieved the totals in Table 10.2 are considered Class 2.

Weight Class (kg)	32	34	38	42	46	50	56	62	69	77	85	94	105	+105
Total (kg)	65	70	80	95	105	120	135	155	170	185	195	205	215	220

Table 10.1 Class 2 Men Qualification

Weight Class (kg)	32	36	40	44	48	53	58	63	69	75	+75
Total (kg)	55	65	75	80	85	95	105	110	115	120	125

Table 10.2 Class 2 Women Qualification

Class 2 lifters are still living their lives as amateurs. The training is not creating such a demand on energy and time resources that the athletes cannot engage in other full-time activities such as employment or meaningful education. The increase in time demands, however, will require improved time management skills and a possible re-inspection of one's personal goals.

The more talented the individual, the less of a problem will be the incorporation of training into the lifestyle. This talent will become more of a factor in terms of the rate of progress. While just about any athlete that has risen to the Class 2 standards will continue to make steady progress in competitive totals, the exceptionally talented athlete will often make dramatic gains without seeming to register any undue stresses in physiological functioning.

This can lead to problems in the future as many exceptionally talented athletes will not begin to develop the necessary eating and hygienic habits that will be indispensable in future training progress.

The Class 2 athlete should be developing the psychological skills and mindset to deal with competitive situations. Some psychological maturation is also expected during this phase so that the lifter learns how to prioritize the various facets of life in order to train most effectively. This maturational process is probably best developed by observing it in peers and role models. Again, the development of the psychic environment is largely the role of the coach.

The necessity for General Physical Preparation will be reduced, but some should be incorporated in order to develop and enhance normal competitive instincts. Some GPP is also necessary to aid in the restoration process, as training should place enough demands on the body that restoration is a necessity.

Another point to keep in mind is the fact that Class 2 lifters are as a group more talented and probably more goal oriented than Class 3s. More is known about the training of Class 2 lifters and subsequently more of the established guidelines are better developed and more meaningful. In scouring the available literature, there are firmer figures available regarding the training parameter prescriptions.

Exercise Selection

The number of exercises employed will be fewer, and the fundamental exercises will occupy a larger percentage of the training volume. Whereas Class 3 training programs usually feature one technical lift per session, this number will increase to two and in some cases three for many of the Class 2 workouts.

The exercise selection should reflect the emphasis that is still being placed on perfecting the mastery of technique of the snatch and clean & jerk. Although the fundamental technique should be sound by this time, an emphasis must be placed on further improvement of technique, which should also lead to a more harmonious development for the performance of these lifts.

The 28 Most Appropriate Exercises To Be Included In the Training Program of a Class 2 Lifter:

1) Snatch
2) Clean & Jerk
3) Cleans
4) Jerk Off Rack
5) Hang Snatch (From 3 different heights)
6) Hang Clean (From 3 different heights)
7) Power Snatch
8) Power Clean
9) Power Jerk (Snatch or clean grip, in front of or back of the neck)
10) Snatch Pull (or Extension)
11) Clean Pull (or Extension
12) Back Squat
13) Front Squat
14) Romanian Deadlift
15) Snatch Deadlift (with or without halts)
16) Clean Deadlift (with or without halts)
17) Good Morning (Bent leg and Straight leg)

18) Bench Press
19) Press (Standing and seated)
20) Push Press (Clean & Snatch grip, in front or back of the Neck)
21) Jerk Recovery
22) Jerk Lockout
23) Jerk Support
24) Overhead Squat
25) Squat Snatch Press
26) Abdominal Exercises
27) Hyperextensions
28) Pull-ups

Yearly Loading Parameters and other considerations

The typical annual loading volume for Class 2 weightlifters ranges from 9,000 to 11,000 repetitions. The number of 90 to 100% lifts in the snatch and clean & jerk will range from 200 to 400. The cleans and jerks are counted separately. Whereas the average intensity for Class 3 was in the 65 to 75% range, the range is now elevated to 73% to 77%. The lowest percentage that is counted in the loading is 60% as opposed to the 50% of Class 3. The number of meaningful competitions per year should be 5. The maximum number of hours per week spent in weightlifting training should not exceed 16.

The percentage of the annual load given over to snatching exercises (classic snatch, snatches from the hang, and snatches from blocks) has been found to ideally comprise 16% of the annual volume, while the cleaning and jerking exercises (classic clean & jerk, cleans, cleans from the hang and from blocks, and jerks and power jerks from racks) will ideally comprise 22% of the annual volume.

The number of training weeks, out of 52, should be 45 weeks, made up of 5 9-week macrocycles. The 7 remaining weeks can be divided up into 4 transition weeks, one at the end of each macrocycle except for the last one.

Calculations

To calculate the number of reps in each macrocycle, mesocycle, microcycle and day, we begin with the annual volume of 9,000 reps. If this is divided by 5 (the number of 9-week macrocycles), the number of repetitions per macrocycle is 1800.

The ratio of a preparation mesocycle volume to a pre-competition mesocycle volume for a Class 2 lifter is 1.59:1. With three mesocycles (two of them being preparation), the ratio of the reps is 1.59:1.59:1. This adds up to a total of 4.18. This can be divided into 1800, giving a ratio of 685 reps for the first preparation month, 685 reps for the second

Mesocycle	Week 1	Week 2	Week 3
Prep 1 (1st 3 weeks)	288	219	178
Prep 2 (2nd 3 weeks)	288	219	178
Pre-Comp (Final 3 weeks)	181	138	119

Table 10.3 Class 2 Weekly Volume

preparation month, 430 reps for the pre-competition month.

3-week mesocycles have their volumes divided into microcycles with the following ratio 42%:32%:26%. (Table 10.3 and Graph 10.1)

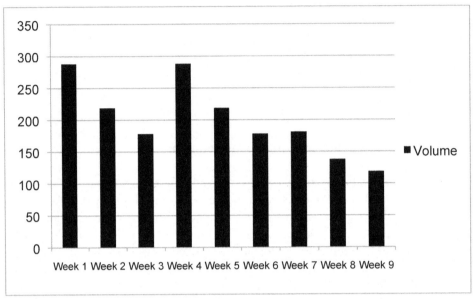

Graph 10.1 Class 2 weekly volume. This represents the distribution of the weekly volumes over the three mesocycles

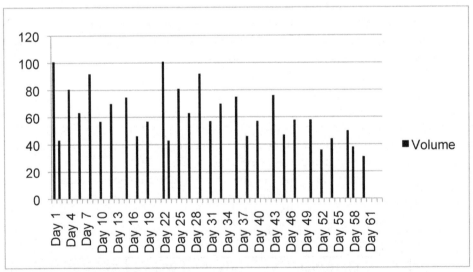

Graph 10.2 Class 2 daily volume. The 1st Prep Mesocycle ends at Day 19. The 2nd Prep Mesocycle ends at Day 40. This represents the daily repetition volume over the entire 9 weeks (63 days) of the Macrocycle. The competition will take place on Day 63.

Week 1 and Week 4 will have four training days, while the rest will have 3 training days. The distribution ratio for a 4-day week is 15%, 22%, 28%, 35%. The distribution ratio for a 3-day week is 26%, 32%, 42%.

Table 10.4 provides the data by which the daily volume graph (Graph 10.2) was calculated. The preceding daily percentages were used to calculate the day volume by multiplying them by the weekly volume. The preparation mesocycle is highlighted in gray.

Table 10.4 Class 2 Daily Volume

Week	Day	Week Vol	Daily %	Day Vol
Week 1	Day 1	288	35%	101
	Day 2		15%	43
	Day 3			
	Day 4		28%	81
	Day 5			
	Day 6		22%	63
	Day 7			
Week 2	Day 8	219	42%	92
	Day 9			
	Day 10		26%	57
	Day 11			
	Day 12		32%	70
	Day 13			
	Day 14			
Week 3	Day 15	178	42%	75
	Day 16			
	Day 17		26%	46
	Day 18			
	Day 19		32%	57
	Day 20			
	Day 21			
Week 4	Day 22	288	35%	101
	Day 23		15%	43
	Day 24			
	Day 25		28%	81
	Day 26			
	Day 27		22%	63
	Day 28			

Week 5	Day 29	219	42%	92
	Day 30			
	Day 31		26%	57
	Day 32			
	Day 33		32%	70
	Day 34			
	Day 35			
Week 6	Day 36	178	42%	75
	Day 37			
	Day 38		26%	46
	Day 39			
	Day 40		32%	57
	Day 41			
	Day 42			
Week 7	Day 43	181	42%	76
	Day 44			
	Day 45		26%	47
	Day 46			
	Day 47		32%	58
	Day 48			
	Day 49			
Week 8	Day 50	138	42%	58
	Day 51			
	Day 52		26%	36
	Day 53			
	Day 54		32%	44
	Day 55			
	Day 56			
Week 9	Day 57	119	42%	50
	Day 58		32%	38
	Day 59			
	Day 60		26%	31
	Day 61			
	Day 62			
	Day 63			

SAMPLE CLASS 2 TRAINING PROGRAM

The numbers to the right represent respectively the number of repetitions in the exercise, the number of repetitions in the workout and the number of repetitions for the week.

Week 1 (Preparation Mesocycle) 287 repetitions

Day 1—Monday (101 repetitions)
1) Snatch: 60%/2, (70%/2)2, (80%/2)2   10:10:10
2) Clean & Jerk: 60%/2+1, (70%/2+1)2, (80%/2+1)2   15:25:25
3) Snatch High Pull: (80%/3)4   12:37:37
4) Back Squat: 60%/3, (70%/3)2, (80%/3)2   15:52:52
5) Power Jerk: 60%/3, 65%/3, (70%/3)2   12:64:64
6) Good Morning: (X/6)4   24:88:88
7) Overhead Squat: 60%/3, (70%/3)4   15:103:103

Day 2—Tuesday (43 repetitions)
1) Power Snatch: 60%/3, 65%/3, (70%/2)3   12:12:115
2) Power Clean & Power Jerk: 60%/3+2, 65%/3+2, (70%/2+2)2   18:30:133
3) Clean Deadlift: (80%/3)4   12:42:145

Day 4—Thursday (81 repetitions)
1) Snatch: 60%/2, 70%/2, (80%/2)3   10:10:155
2) Clean & Jerk: 60%/2+1, 70%/2+1, (80%/2+1)3   15:25:170
3) Snatch Extension: (80%/3)4   12:37:182
4) Front Squat: 60%/3, 70%/3, 75%/3, (80%/3)2   15:52:197
5) Behind the Neck Push Press: 60%/4, 65%/4, (70%/3)2   14:66:211
6) Squat Snatch Press: (X/4)4   16:82:227

Day 6—Saturday (63 repetitions)
1) Power Snatch & Overhead Squat: 60%/3+3, (65%/3+3)2, (70%/3+3)2   30:30:257
2) Power Clean & Power Jerk: 60%/3+3, (65%/3+3)2, (70%/3+3)2   30:60:287

Week 2 (Preparation Mesocycle) 219 repetitions

Day 8—Monday (92 repetitions)
1) Snatch: 60%/2, 70%/2, (80%/2)4   12:12:12
2) Power Clean & Jerk: 60%/2+2, 65%/2+2, (70%/2+2)2   16:28:28
3) Clean Deadlift: 80%/4, (85%/3)3   13:41:41
4) Back Squat: 60%/4, (70%/4)2, (80%/3)2   18:59:59
5) Press: (X/4)4   16:75:75
6) Good Morning: (X/4)4   16:91:91

Day 10—Wednesday (57 repetitions)
1) Power Snatch: 60%/2, 65%/2, (70%/2)3   10:10:101
2) Clean: 60%/3, (70%/3)2, (80%/3)2   15:25:116
3) Snatch High Pull: (80%/4)4   16:41:132
4) Back Squat: 60%/4, (70%/4)2, 75%/4   16:57:148

Day 12—Friday (70 repetitions)
1) Snatch: 60%/3, (70%/3)2, (80%/3)2   15:15:163
2) Hang Power Clean: 60%/4, (65%/3)2, (70%/3)2   16:31:179
3) Jerk off Rack: 60%/3, (70%/3)2, (80%/3)2   15:46:194
4) Clean Extension: (80%/4)4   16:60:210
5) Bench Press: (X/3)3   09:69:219

Week 3 (Preparation Mesocycle) 178 Repetitions

Day 15—Monday (75 repetitions)
1) Power Snatch: 60%/3, (65%/3)2, (70%/3)2   15:15:15
2) Clean & Jerk: 60%/1+3, (70%/1+3)2, (80%/1+2)2   18:33:33
3) Snatch Extension: (85%/3)4   12:45:45
4) Front Squat: 60%/3, (70%/3)2, (80%/3)2   15:60:60
5) Press: (X/3)5   15:75:75

Day 17--Wednesday (46 repetitions)
1) Snatch: 60%/2, 70%/2, 75%/2, 80%/2   08:08:83
2) Power Clean: 60%/3, 65%/3, (70%/3)2   12:20:95
3) Back Squat: 60%/3, 70%/3, 80%/3, 85%/2   11:31:106
4) Clean Extension: (80%/3)5   15:46:121

Day 19--Friday (57 repetitions)
1) Hang Power Snatch: 60%/3, (65%/3)2, (70%/3)2   15:15:136
2) Clean & Jerk: 60%/3+1, (70%/3+1)2, (80%/3+1)2   20:35:156
3) Back Squat: 60%/4, 70%/4, (80%/3)3   17:52:173

Week 4 (Preparation Mesocycle) 288 repetitions

Day 22--Monday (101 repetitions)
1) Hang Snatch: 60%/3, (70%/3)2, (80%/3)3   18:18:18
2) Power Clean: 60%/4, (65%/4)2, (70%/3)2   18:36:36
3) Behind the Neck Power Jerk: 60%/4, (65%/4)2, (70%/3)2   18:54:54
4) Snatch Extension: (80%/4)4   16:70:70
5) Front Squat: 60%/4, (70%/4)2, (80%/4)2   20:90:90
6) Bench Press: (X/3)4   12:102:102

Day 23—Tuesday (43 repetitions)
1) Power Snatch: 60%/2, (65%/2)2, (70%/2)2   10:10:112
2) Clean: 60%/4, (70%/4)2, (80%/3)2   18:28:130
3) Power Jerk: 60%/3, (65%/3)2, (70%/3)2   15:43:145

Day 25—Thursday (81 repetitions)
1) Snatch: 60%/2, 70%/2, 80%/2, (85%/2)2   10:10:155
2) Power Clean & Power Jerk: 60%/3+3, (65%/3+3)2, (70%/3+3)2   30:40:185
3) Clean Deadlift: (85%/4)4   16:56:201
4) Back Squat: 60%/4, (70%/4)2, (80%/4)2   20:76:221
5) Press: (X/2)4   08:84:229

Day 27—Saturday (63 repetitions)
1) Power Snatch & Overhead Squat: 60%/3+3, (65%/3+3)2, (70%/3+3)2 30:30:259
2) Clean: 60%/2, 70%/2, 80%/2, 85%/2   08:38:267
3) Snatch High Pull: (80%/4)4   16:54:283
4) Back Squat: 60%/2, 70%/2, 80%/2, 85%/2   08:62:291

Week 5 (Preparation Mesocycle) 219 repetitions

Day 29—Monday (92 repetitions)
1) Snatch: 60%/3, 70%/3, 80%/3, 85%/2, (80%/3)2   17:17:17
2) Hang Power Clean: 60%/3, 65%/3, (70%/302   12:29:29
3) Power Jerk: 60%/3, 65%/3, (70%/3)2   12:41:41
4) Clean Extension: (80%/3)2, (85%/2)2   10:51:51
5) Back Squat: 60%/3, 70%/3, (80%/3)2, (85%/2)2   16:67:67
6) Good Morning: (X/6)4   24:91:91

Day 31—Wednesday (57 repetitions)
1) Hang Power Snatch: 60%/3, 65%/3, (70%/3)2   12:12:103
2) Clean & Jerk: 60%/3+1, 70%/3+1, (80%/3+1)2   16:28:119
3) Snatch High Pull: (85%/3)4   12:40:131
4) Front Squat: 60%/3, 70%/3, (80%/3)3   15:55:146

Day 33—Friday (70 repetitions)
1) Snatch: 60%/2, 70%/2, (80%/2)2, 85%/2   10:10:156
2) Cleans: 60%/2, 70%/2, (80%/2)3   10:20:166
3) Jerk off Rack: 60%/2, 70%/2, (80%/2)3   10:30:176
4) Romanian Deadlift: (85%/3)4   12:42:188
5) Back Squat: 60%/4, (70%/4)2, (80%/4)2   20:62:208
6) Press: (X/3)4   12:74:221

Week 6 (Preparation Mesocycle) 178 repetitions

Day 36—Monday (75 repetitions)
1) Hang Power Snatch: 60%/3, 65%/3, (70%/3)2   12:12:12
2) Power Clean & Power Jerk: 60%/3+2, 65%/3+2, (70%/2+2)2   18:30:30
3) Snatch Extension: (80%/4)4   16:46:46
4) Back Squat: 60%/4, (70%/4)2, 80%/4, 85%/2, 80%/4   22:68:68
5) Press: (X/2)4   08:76:76

Day 38—Wednesday (46 repetitions)
1) Snatch: 60%/2, 70%/2, 80%/2, 85%/2, 90%/1   09:09:85
2) Clean & Jerk: 60%/2+2, 70%/2+2, 80%/2+2, 85%/2+1, 90%/1+1   17:26:97
3) Clean Extension: (90%/2)4   08:34:105
4) Front Squat: 60%/2, 70%/2, 80%/2, 85%/2, (90%/2)2   12:46:117

Day 40—Friday (57 repetitions)
1)Power Snatch: 60%/3, 65%/3, (70%/3)3   15:15:132
2)Power Clean: 60%/3, 65%/3, (70%/3)3   15:30:147
3)Power Jerk: 60%/2, (70%/2)3   08:38:155
4)Back Squat: 60%/3, 70%/3, 80%/3, 85%/3, 90%/1 13:51:168
5)Press: (X/2)3   06:57:174

Week 7 (Pre-Competition Mesocycle) 181 Repetitions

Day 43—Monday (76 repetitions)
1) Snatch: 60%/2, 70%/2, 80%/2, 85%/2, 90%/1, 80%/2, 85%/2, 90%/1   14:14:14
2) Clean & Jerk: 60%/2+1, 70%/2+1, 80%/2+1, 85%/2+1,
        90%/1+1, 80%/2+1, 85%/2+1, 90%/1+1   22:36:36
3) Snatch Extension: (90%/2)4   08:44:44
4) Front Squat: 60%/3, 70%/3, 80%/3, 85%/3, 90%/2, 80%/3, 85%/2   19:63:63
5) Press: (X/3)4   12:75:75

Day 45—Wednesday (47 repetitions)
1) Power Snatch: 60%/2, 65%/2, 70%/2, 75%/1, 65%/2, 70%/2   11:11:86
2) Power Clean & Jerk: 60%/2+1, 65%/2+1, 70%/2+1,
        75%/1+1, 65%/2+1, 70%/2+1   17:28:103
3) Clean High Pull: (85%/3)4   12:40:115
4) Back Squat: 60%/2, 70%/2, 80%/2, 85%/2   08:48:123

Day 47—Friday (58 repetitions)
1) Snatch: 60%/2, 70%/2, (80%/2)2   08:08:131
2) Clean & Jerk: 60%/2+1, 70%/2+1, (80%/2+1)2   12:20:143
3) Snatch High Pull: (90%/2)4   08:28:151
4) Back Squat: 60%/1, 70%/1, 80%/1, (85%/3)3   12:40:163
5) Good Morning: (X/5)4   20:60:183

Week 8 (Pre-Competition Mesocycle) 138 repetitions

Day 50—Monday (58 repetitions)
1) Snatch: 60%/1, 70%/1, 80%/1, 85%/1, 90%/1, 95%/1, 85%/1, 90%/1   08:08:08
2) Clean & Jerk: 60%/1+1, 70%/1+1, 80%/1+1, 85%/1+1,
        90%/1+1, 95%/1+1, 85%/1+1, 90%/1+1   16:24:24
3) Front Squat: 60%/2, 70%/2, 80%/2, 85%/2, 90%/2, 95%/1, 90%/2   13:37:37
4) Clean Extension: (90%/2)4   08:45:45
5) Push Press: 60%/3, 65%/3, (70%/2)3   12:57:57

Day 52—Wednesday (36 repetitions)
1) Power Snatch: 60%/2, 65%/2, 70%/2, 75%/1, 70%/2   09:09:66
2) Power Clean & Power Jerk: 60%/2+1, 65%/2+1,
        70%/2+1, 75%/1+1, 70%/2+1   14:23:80
3) Back Squat: 60%2/ 70%/2, 80%/2, 85%/2, 90%/2, (95%/1)2 12:35:92

Day 54—Friday (44 repetitions)
1) Snatch: 60%/1, 70%/1, 80%/1, 85%/1, 90%/1, 85%/1, 90%/1   07:07:99
2) Clean & Jerk: 60%/1+1, 70%/1+1, 80%/1+1,
    85%/1+1, 90%/1+1, 85%/1+1, 90%/1+1   14:21:113
3) Front Squat: 60%/2, 70%/2, 80%/2, 90%/2, 95%/1, 90%/2, 95%/1   12:33:125
4) Snatch High Pull: (95%/2)4   08:41:133

Week 9 (Pre-competition Mesocycle) (119 reps)

Day 57—Monday (50 reps)
1) Snatch: 60%/1, 70%/1, 80%/1, (85%/1)3   06:06:06
2) Clean & Jerk: 60%/1+1, 70%/1+1, 80%/1+1, (85%/1+1)3   12:18:18
3) Snatch High Pull: (90%/2)4   08:26:26
4) Front Squat: 60%/2, 70%/2, 80%/2, 85%/2, 90%/1, 85%/2   11:37:37
5) Press: (X/3)4   12:49:49

Day 58—Tuesday (38 reps)
1) Power Snatch: 60%/1, 65%/1, 70%/1, 75%/1, 70%/1   05:05:54
2) Power Clean & Jerk: 60%/1+1, 65%/1+1, 70%/1+1,
    75%/1+1, 70%/1+1   10:15:64
3) Clean High Pull: 80%/2, 85%/2, 90%/1, 80%/2   07:22:71
4) Back Squat: 60%/3, 70%/3, 80%/3, 85%/2   11:33:82

Day 60—Thursday, (31 reps)
1) Power Snatch: 60%/2, (65%/2)2   06:06:88
2) Power Clean & Jerk: 60%/2+2, (65%/2+2)2   12:18:100
3) Jumping Back Squat: (50%/3)3   09:27:109
4) Press: (X/3)3   09:36:118

CHAPTER 11
CLASS 1 TRAINING

Class 1 lifters are in the upper reaches of the avid hobbyist stage. They are at a point in their development where their technique is highly refined. Their speed characteristics, if not highly developed, are approaching their ultimate levels. They are beginning to be in need of periodic dedicated restoration. They are performing less GPP. Hygienic and nutritional factors play a larger role in the training process.

Male weightlifters who have achieved the totals in Table 1.1 are considered Class 1. Female weightlifters who have achieved the totals in Table 1.2 are considered Class 1.

Weight Class (kg)	56	62	69	77	85	94	105	+105
Total (kg)	155	175	190	210	225	235	240	245

Table 11.1 Class 1 Male Qualification

Weight Class (kg)	48	53	58	63	69	75	+75
Total (kg)	95	105	115	120	130	135	140

Table 11.2 Class 1 Women Qualification

As far as training is concerned, a Class 1 weightlifter should be used to the periodized nature of training. He or she should have developed an understanding of the training cycles, and the proper approach to take toward missed lifts, and the difficulty experienced during the critical parts of the preparation cycle.

The talent of an athlete will begin to show through while undergoing the Class 1 training regimen. The training loads have become sufficient to adversely affect the speed of movement of a less talented athlete. The more talented athlete will experience much less of a speed loss during the more demanding weeks of the preparation mesocycle.

Exercise Selection

The exercises to be employed are much smaller in number than they were for Classes 3 and 2. They are more geared toward developing strength in an individual who has been trained to be balanced for the execution of the snatch and clean & jerk. There will be fewer pulling movements performed from the various hang heights and from blocks. There will be fewer partial movements, and the exact selection will be to remediate areas that are stubbornly resistant to previous efforts to bring about a balanced development.

The variety of exercises and their variants will be much greater during the preparation mesocycles, and the intensities will be increased during the pre-competition mesocycle.

The 18 Most Appropriate Exercises To Be Included In the Training Program of a Class 1 Lifter:

1) Snatch
2) Clean & Jerk
3) Cleans
4) Jerk off Rack
5) Power Snatch
6) Power Clean
7) Power Jerk
8) Snatch Pull (or Extension)
9) Clean Pull (or Extension)
10) Snatch Deadlift
11) Clean Deadlift
12) Romanian Deadlift
13) Back Squat
14) Front Squat
15) Push Press
16) Press
17) Good Mornings
18) Overhead Squat

Yearly Loading Parameters

The following numbers were determined by studying the training of classified lifters as they progressed through the Sport School program of the Soviet Union. They are guideline figures to provide some direction for assembling the training program. The developing coach should not put forth an extended effort to try and make sure that all the numbers fit. Approximations that represent the proper trends are sufficient.

The typical annual loading volume for Class 1 weightlifters is in the 11,000 to 13,000 repetition range. The number of 90%—100% repetitions is in the 200—400 range, and the relative intensity in the snatch and clean & jerk exercises remains in the 73% to 77% range. The number of meaningful competitions is best set at 4 to 5. The best percentages of snatch lifts and clean & jerk lifts in training has been established as 18% and 22% respectively. Snatch and clean & jerk exercises refer specifically to classic snatches and classic cleans, power snatches and power cleans, and classic jerks and power jerks.

The average volume for a four-week preparation mesocycle is 1,424, while the same figure for a four week pre-competition mesocycle is 908. During the preparation mesocycle, the number of 90%—100% repetitions in snatches and cleans & jerks is 44 and during the pre-competition Mesocycle is 56.

Loading in Zones of Intensity: Distribution of Year Volume

The percentages in Table 11.3 represent the percentage of the annual repetitions for the exercise group designated in the first column. All of these numbers have been empirically derived and represent trends. Some deviations from these figures is acceptable and actually necessary to deal with individual situations.

Intensity	50-55%	60-65%	70-75%	80-85%	90-95%	100-105%	110%	Yearly Average
Snatch		7%	56%	28%	8%	1%		75%
Clean & Jerk		4%	45%	39%	11%	1%		77%
Snatch Pull				24%	33%	39%	4%	92%
Clean Pull			17%	34%	26%	19%	4%	84%
Squats	14%	27%	21%	35%	3%			70%
Fundamental Exercises*	3%	11%	31%	31%	16%	7%	1%	78%

Table 11.3 Class 1 Zones of Intensity
These are exercises from Groups 1—10 in Chapter 8

It is also important to keep in mind that there will be occasional competitions that lie without the normal peaking procedure of the macrocycle. It may be necessary at times to adjust a specific week's training characteristics to accommodate the competition date, while still maintaining the direction and theme of the given mesocycle. This is a planning skill that coaches must master in order to maintain the integrity of the training cycles.

Calculations

An optimal macrocycle should be composed of two preparation mesocycles and one pre-competition mesocycle. This may or may not be followed by a one-week transitional microcycle.

For a mesocycle of more than 1000 reps, the weeks work well with the following percentages: 30%, 27%, 23% and 20%, though not necessarily in this order.

For a mesocycle of less than 1000 reps, the weeks work well with the following percentages 35%, 28%, 22%, 15% though not necessarily in this order. (Tables 11.4 and Graph 11.1)

Prep Month 1	Week 1	Week 2	Week 3	Week 4
Volume	427	327	384	285
Prep Month 2	Week 5	Week 6	Week 7	Week 8
Volume	427	384	327	285
Pre-Competition	Week 9	Week 10	Week 11	Week 12
Volume	317	254	200	136

Table 11.4 Class 1 Weekly Volume

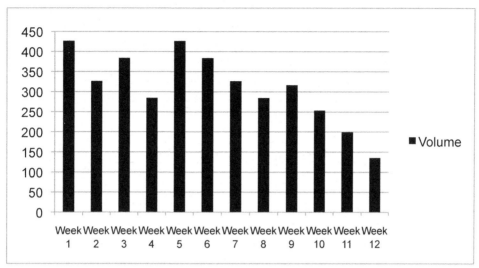

Graph 11.1 Class 1 weekly volume. A 12-Week Class 1 Macrocycle showing weekly volumes

Week	1	2	3	4	5	6	7	8	9	10	11	12
Training Days	5	4	5	4	5	5	4	4	4	4	3	3

Table 11.5 Class 1 Training Days per Week

Table 11.6 provides the data by which the daily volume graph (Graph 11.2) was calculated. The daily volumes were calculated by multiplying the weekly volume by the daily volume percentage. The preparation mesocycle is highlighted in gray.

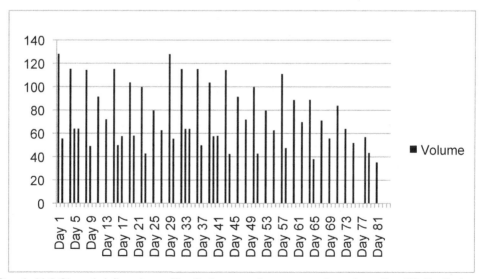

Graph 11.2 Class 1 daily volume. The first preparation mesocycle ends on Day 28, the 2nd one ends on Day 56. The Pre-competition mesocycle runs from Day 57 to Day 84.

Table 11.6 Class 1 Daily Volume

Week	Day	Week Vol	Daily %	Day Vol
Week 1	Day 1	427	30%	128
	Day 2		13%	56
	Day 3			
	Day 4		27%	115
	Day 5		15%	64
	Day 6		15%	64
	Day 7			
Week 2	Day 8	327	35%	114
	Day 9		15%	49
	Day 10			
	Day 11		28%	92
	Day 12			
	Day 13		22%	72
	Day 14			
Week 3	Day 15	384	30%	115
	Day 16		13%	50
	Day 17		15%	58
	Day 18			
	Day 19		27%	104
	Day 20		15%	58
	Day 21			
Week 4	Day 22	285	35%	100
	Day 23		15%	43
	Day 24			
	Day 25		28%	80
	Day 26			
	Day 27		22%	63
	Day 28			
Week 5	Day 29	427	30%	128
	Day 30		13%	56
	Day 31			
	Day 32		27%	115
	Day 33		15%	64
	Day 34		15%	64
	Day 35			

Week 6	Day 36	384	30%	115
	Day 37		13%	50
	Day 38			
	Day 39		27%	104
	Day 40		15%	58
	Day 41		15%	58
	Day 42			
Week 7	Day 43	327	35%	114
	Day 44		13%	43
	Day 45			
	Day 46		28%	92
	Day 47			
	Day 48		22%	72
	Day 49			
Week 8	Day 50	285	35%	100
	Day 51		15%	43
	Day 52			
	Day 53		28%	80
	Day 54			
	Day 55		22%	63
	Day 56			
Week 9	Day 57	317	35%	111
	Day 58		15%	48
	Day 59			
	Day 60		28%	89
	Day 61			
	Day 62		22%	70
	Day 63			
Week 10	Day 64	254	35%	89
	Day 65		15%	38
	Day 66			
	Day 67		28%	71
	Day 68			
	Day 69		22%	56
	Day 70			

Week 11	Day 71	200	42%	84
	Day 72			
	Day 73		32%	64
	Day 74			
	Day 75		26%	52
	Day 76			

SAMPLE CLASS 1 TRAINING PROGRAM

The numbers to the right represent respectively the number of repetitions in the exercise, the number of repetitions in the workout and the number of repetitions for the week.

Week 1 (Preparation Mesocycle) 427 repetitions

Day 1—Monday (128 repetitions)
1) Snatch: 60%/2, (70%/2)3, (75%/2)2   12:12:12
2) Clean & Jerk: 60%/2+2, (70%/2+2)3, (75%/2+2)2   24:36:36
3) Snatch Extension: (80%/3)4   12:48:48
4) Clean Deadlift: (80%/4)4   16:64:64
5) Back Squat: 60%/3, (70%/3)3, (75%/3)2   18:82:82
6) Push Press: (60%/3)2, (65%/3)2, (70%/2)2   16:98:98
7) Good Morning: (X/7)4   28:126:126

Day 2—Tuesday (56 repetitions
1) Power Snatch: 60%/3, 65%/3, (70%/3)2   12:12:138
2) Power Clean: 60%/3, 65%/3, (70%/3)2   12:24:150
3) Snatch Deadlift: (90%/4)4   16:40:166
4) Behind the Neck Power Jerk: 60%/4, 65%/4, (70%/4)2   16:56:182

Day 4—Thursday (115 repetitions)
1) Snatch: 60%/3, 70%/3, (80%/2)3   12:12:194
2) Clean & Jerk: 60%/2+2, 70%/2+2, (80%/2+2)2   16:28:210
3) Clean High Pull: (90%/4)4   16:42:226
4) Snatch Deadlift: (95%/4)4   16:58:242
4) Front Squat: 60%/3, (70%/3)3, (80%/2)2   16:74:258
5)Push Press: (60%/3)2, (65%/3)2, (70%/3)2   18:92:276
6) Good Morning: (X/6)4   24:116:300

Day 5—Friday (64 repetitions)
1) Power Snatch & Overhead Squat: 60%/3+3, 65%/3+3, (70%/3+3)2   24:24:324
2) Power Clean & Power Jerk: 60%/3+3, 65%/3+3, (70%/3+3)2   24:48:348
3) Romanian Deadlift: (85%/4)4   16:64:364

Day 6—Saturday (64 repetitions)
1) Snatch: 60%/2, 70%/2, (80%/2)3   10:10:374
2) Clean & Jerk: 60%/2+1, 70%/2+1, (80%/2+1)3   15:25:389
3) Snatch Extension: (90%/3)4   12:37:401
4) Back Squat: 60%/3, 70%/3, (80%/3)3   15:52:416
5) Behind the Neck Jerk Off Rack: (80%/3)4   12:64:428

Week 2 (Preparation Mesocycle) 327 repetitions

Day 8—Monday (114 repetitions)
1) Snatch: 60%/4, 70%/4, (80%/3)3   17:17:17
2) Clean & Jerk: 60%/4+1, 70%/4+1, (80%/3+1)3   22:39:39
3) Jerk off Rack: 70%/3, (80%/3)3   12:51:51
4) Snatch High Pull: (85%/3)2, (90%/3)2   12:63:63
5) Back Squat: 60%/4, 70%/4, (80%/3)3   17:80:80
6) Romanian Deadlift: (85%/4)4   16:96:96
7) Push Press: 60%/4, 65%/4, (70%/4)2   16:112:112

Day 9—Tuesday (49 repetitions0
1) Power Snatch & Overhead Squat: 60%/3+3, 65%/3+3, (70%/3+3)2   24:24:136
2) Power Clean & Power Jerk: 60%/3+3, 65%/3+3, (70%/3+3)2   24:48:160

Day 11—Thursday (92 repetitions)
1) Hang Snatch: 60%/3, (70%/3)2, (80%/3)2   15:15:175
2) Hang Clean: 60%/4, (70%/4)2, (80%/3)2   18:33:193
3) Clean Extension: (85%/4)4   16:49:209
4) Front Squat: 60%/4, (70%/4)2, (80%/3)3   21:70:230
5) Push Press: 60%/4, (65%/4)2, (70%/4)2   20:90:250

Day 13—Saturday (72 repetitions)
1) Power Snatch: 60%/4, (65%/4)2, (70%/4)2   20:20:270
2) Hang Power Clean: 60%/4, (65%/4)2, (70%/4)2   20:40:290
3) Snatch High Pull: (80%/4)2, (90%/4)2   16:56:306
4) Press: (X/5)4   20:76:326

Week 3 (Preparation Mesocycle) 384 repetitions

Day 15—Monday (115 repetitions)
1) Snatch: 60%/4, 70%/4, 80%/4, (80%/3)2   18:18:18
2) Cleans: 60%/4, 70%/4, 80%/4, (80%/3)2   18:36:36
3) Jerk off rack: 70%/4, (80%/4)4   20:56:56
4) Clean High Pull: (80%/4)2, (85%/4)2, (90%/3)2   22:78:78
5) Back Squat: 60%/4, 70%/4, (80%/4)4   24:102:102
6) Press: (X/3)4   12:114:114

Day 16—Tuesday (50 repetitions)
1) Hang Power Snatch: 60%/4, 65%/4, (70%/4)3   20:20:134
2) Hang Power Clean: 60%/4, 65%/4, (70%/4)3   20:40:154
3) Snatch Extension: (90%/2)5   10:50:164

Day 17—Wednesday (58 repetitions)
1) Snatch High Pull & Snatch: 60%/3+1, 70%/3+1, (80%/3+1)3   20:20:184
2) Clean High Pull & Clean: 60%/3+1, 70%/3+1, (80%/3+1)3   20:40:204
3) Front Squat: 60%/3, 70%/3, (80%/3)4   18:58:222

Day 19—Friday (104 repetitions)
1) Snatch: 60%/3, 70%/3, 80%/3, (85%/2)3   15:15:237
2) Clean & Jerk: 60%/3+2, 70%/3+2, 80%/3+2, (85%/2+2)3   27:42:264
3) Clean Extension: (90%/3)4   12:54:276
4) Romanian Deadlift: (85%/4)5   20:74:296
5) Back Squat: 60%/3, 70%/3, 80%/3, (85%/3)2, 80%/3   18:92:314
6) Press: (X/3)4   12:104:326

Day 20—Saturday (58 repetitions)
1) Power Snatch: 60%/2, 65%/2, (70%/2)3   10:10:336
2) Power Clean & Power Jerk: 60%/2+2, 65%/2+2, (70%/2+2)3   20:30:356
3) Snatch Extension: (85%/3)4   12:42:368
4) Push Press: 60%/4, 65%/4, (70%/4)2   16:58:384

Week 4 (Preparation Mesocycle) 285 Repetitions

Day 22—Monday (100 repetitions)
1) Snatch: 60%/4, 70%/4, (80%/4)3   20:20:20
2) Clean & Jerk: 60%/4+1, 70%/4+1, (80%/4+1)3   25:45:45
3) Snatch High Pull: (85%/4)4   16:61:61
4) Jerk off Rack: 70%/3, (80%/3)2, 85%/2   14:75:75
5) Back Squat: 60%/4, 70%/4, (80%/4)4   24:99:99

Day 23—Tuesday (43 repetitions)
1) Power Snatch: 60%/3, 65%/3, (70%/3)3   15:15:114
2) Power Clean & Power Jerk: 60%/3+3, 65%/3+3, (70%/3+3)3   30:45:144

Day 25—Thursday (80 repetitions)
1) Snatch: 60%/3, 70%/3, (80%/3)3   15:15:159
2) Clean: 60%/3, 70%/3, (80%/3)3   15:30:174
3) Clean Extension: (85%/4)4   16:46:190
4) Front Squat: 60%/4, 70%/4, (80%/4)3   20:66:210
5) Push Press: 60%/4, 65%/4, (70%/3)2   14:80:224

Day 26—Friday (63 repetitions)
1) Power Snatch & Overhead Squat: 60%/3+3, 65%/3+3, (70%/3+3)3   30:30:254
2) Hang Power Clean: 60%/4, 65%/4, (70%/3)3   17:47:271
3) Back Squat: 60%/3, 70%/3, (80%/3)3   15:62:283

Week 5 (Preparation Mesocycle) 427 Repetitions

Day 29—Monday (128 repetitions)
1) Snatch: 60%/4, 70%/4, (80%/4)4   24:24:24
2) Clean: 60%/4, 70%/4, (80%/4)4   24:48:48
3) Jerk off Rack: 60%/3, 70%/3, (80%/3)2, (85%/3)2   18:66:66
4) Snatch High Pull: (85%/4)4   16:82:82
5) Back Squat: 60%/4, 70%/4, (80%/4)4   24:106:106
6) Press: (X/4)5   20:126:126

Day 30—Tuesday (56 repetitions)
1) Power Snatch: 60%/4, 65%/4, (70%/4)3   20:20:146
2) Power Clean & Jerk: 60%/4+2, 65%/4+2, (70%/4+2)3   30:50:176
3) Clean Deadlift: (90%/2)4   08:58:184

Day 32—Thursday (115 repetitions)
1) Snatch High Pull & Snatch: 60%/3+1, 70%/3+1, (80%/3+1)3   20:20:204
2) Clean High Pull & Clean: 60%/3+1, 70%/3+1, (80%/3+1)3   20:40:224
3) Jerk off Rack: 60%/3, 70%/3, (80%/3)2, (85%/3)2   18:58:242
4) Romanian Deadlift: (85%/4)4   16:74:258
5) Front Squat: 60%/4, 70%/4, (80%/4)4   24:100:282
6) Push Press: 60%/4, 65%/4, (70%/4)2   16:116:298

Day 33—Friday (64 repetitions)
1) Hang Power Snatch: 60%/3, 65%/3, (70%/3)3   15:15:313
2) Hang Power Clean: 60%/3, 65%/3, (70%/3)3   15:30:328
3) Behind the Neck Power Jerk: 60%/3, 65%/3, 70%/3, 75%/2, 70%/3 14:44:342
4) Snatch High Pull: (85%/4)5   20:64:362

Day 34—Saturday (64 repetitions)
1) Snatch: 60%/3, 70%/3, (80%/3)3   15:15:377
2) Clean & Jerk: 60%/2+2, 70%/2+2, (80%/2+2)3   20:35:397
3) Clean Extension: (85%/4)4   16:51:413
4) Back Squat: 60%/3, 70%/3, (80%/3)2   12:63:425

Week 6 (Preparation Mesocycle) 384 repetitions

Day 36—Monday (115 repetitions)
1) Hang Snatch: 60%/3, 70%/3, (80%/3)4   18:18:18
2) Hang Clean: 60%/3, 70%/3, (80%/3)3   15:33:33
3) Snatch Extension: (85%/4)4   16:49:49
4) Back Squat: 60%/4, 70%/4, (80%/4, 85%/1)3   23:62:62
5) Behind the Neck Power Jerk: 60%/3, (70%/3)2 (75%/3)3   18:80:80
6) Romanian Deadlift: (85%/4)5   20:100:100
7) Press: (X/4)4   16:116:116

Day 37—Tuesday (50 repetitions)
1) Power Snatch: 60%/2, 65%/2, (70%/2)2   08:08:124
2) Power Clean: 60%/2+2, 65%/2+2, (70%/2+2)2   16:24:140
3) Clean High Pull: (80%/3)2, (90%/3)2   12:36:152
4) Push Press: 60%/3, 65%/3, (70%/3)3   15:51:167

Day 39—Thursday (104 repetitions)
1) Snatch: 60%/4, 70%/4, (80%/4, 85%/1)3   23:23:190
2) Clean: 60%/4, 70%/4, (80%/4, 85%/1)3   23:46:213
3) Jerk off Rack: 60%/4, 70%/4, (80%/4)2, (85%/2)2   20:66:233
4) Snatch High Pull: (90%/4)4   16:82:249
5) Front Squat: 60%/4, 70%/4, (80%/4, 85%/1)3   23:105:272

Day 40—Friday (58 repetitions)
1) Power Snatch & Behind the Neck Push Press & Overhead Squat:
    60%/3+3+3, 65%/3+3+3, (70%/3+3+3)2   36:36:308
2) Power Clean & Front Squat & Power Jerk:
    60%/3+3+3, 65%/3+3+3, 70%/2+2+2   24:60:332

Day 41—Saturday (58 repetitions)
1) Snatch: 60%/2, 70%/2, (80%/2)2   08:08:340
2) Clean & Jerk: 60%/2+2, 70%/2+2, (80%/2+2)2   16:24:356
3) Clean Extension: (90%/3)4   12:36:368
4) Back Squat: 60%/3, 70%/3, 80%/3, (85%/3)3   18:54:386

Week 7 (Preparation Mesocycle) 327 repetitions

Day 43—Monday (114) repetitions
1) Snatch: 60%/4, 70%/4, (80%/4)4   24:24:24
2) Clean & Jerk: 60%/4+1, 70%/4+1, (80%/4+1)4   30:54:54
3) Jerk off Rack: (80%/3)3   09:63:63
4) Back Squat: 60%/4, 70%/4, (80%/4)4   24:87:87
5) Snatch Extension: (95%/4)4   16:103:103
6) Press: (X/3)4   12:115:115

Day 44—Tuesday (43 repetitions)
1) Power Snatch: 60%/3, 65%/3, (70%/3)2, (75%/2)2   16:16:131
2) Power Clean & Power Jerk:
    60%/3+3, 65%/3+3, (70%/3+2)2, (75%/2+1)2   28:44:159

Day 46—Thursday (92 repetitions)
1) Snatch: 60%/3, 70%/3, 80%/3, (85%/3)3   18:18:178
2) Clean & Jerk: 60%/3+1, 70%/3+1, 80%/3+1, (85%/3+1)3   24:42:202
3) Clean Extension: (95%/3)4   12:54:214
4) Front Squat: 60%/4, 70%/4, (80%/4)4   24:78:238
5) Push Press: 60%/4, 65%/4, (70%/4)2   16:93:254

Day 48—Saturday (72 repetitions)
1) Power Snatch & Overhead Squat: 60%/1+3, 65%/1+3, (70%/1+3)3   20:20:274
2) Power Clean & Power Jerk: 60%/1+3, 65%/1+3, (70%/1+3)3   20:40:294
3) Snatch High Pull: (90%/3)5   15:55:309
4) Back Squat: 60%/3, 70%/3, (80%/3)2, (85%/3)2   18:73:327

Week 8 (Preparation Mesocycle) 285 repetitions

Day 50—Monday (100 repetitions)
1) Snatch: 60%/3, 70%/3, 80%/3, (85%/3)4   21:21:21
2) Clean & Jerk: 60%/3+1, 70%/3+1, 80%/3+1, (85%/3+1)4   28:49:49
3) Clean High Pull: (90%/4)4   16:65:65
4) Back Squat: 60%/3, 70%/3, 80%/3, (85%/3)4   21:86:86
5) Power Jerk: 60%/3, 65%/3, (70%/3)3   15:101:101

Day 51—Tuesday (43 repetitions)
1) Power Snatch: 60%/2, 65%/2, (70%/2)3   10:10:111
2) Power Clean & Power Jerk: 60%/2+2, 65%/2+2, (70%/2+2)3   20:30:131
3) Snatch Extension: (95%/3)4   12:42:143

Day 53—Thursday (80 repetitions)
1) Snatch: 60%/2, 70%/2, 80%/2, (85%/2)4   14:14:157
2) Clean & Jerk: 60%/2+1, 70%/2+1, 80%/2+1, (85%/2+1)4   21:35:179
3) Clean Extension: (90%/3)2, (95%/3)3   15:50:194
4) Front Squat: 60%/3, 70%/3, 80%/3, (85%/3)4   21:71:215
5) Press: (X/3)4   12:83:227

Day 55—Saturday (63 repetitions)
1) Power Snatch: 60%/2, 65%/2, (70%/2)2, (75%/2)2   12:12:239
2) Power Clean & Power Jerk:
      60%/2+2, 65%/2+2, (70%/2+2)2, (75%/2+2)2   24:36:263
3) Snatch High Pull: (100%/3)4   12:48:275
4) Back Squat: 60%/3, 70%/3, (80%/3)2, 85%/3   15:63:290

Week 9 (Pre-competition Mesocycle) 317 repetitions

Day 57—111 repetitions
1) Snatch: 60%/1, 70%/1, 80%/1, 85%/1, 90%/1, 80%/1,
      85%/1, 90%/1, (80%/3)3   17:17:17
2) Clean & Jerk: 60%/1+1, 70%/1+1, 80%/1+1, 85%/1+1,
      90%/1+1, 80%/1+1, 85%/1+1, 90%/1+1, (80%/3+1)3   28:45:45
3) Snatch Extension: (100%/2)4   08:53:53
4) Power Jerk: 70%/3, (75%/3)2, (80%/2)2   13:66:66
5) Front Squat: 60%/1, 70%/1, 80%/1, 85%/1, 90%/1,
      80%/1, 85%/1, 90%/1, (80%/3)4   20:86:86
6) Clean Deadlift: (95%/3)4   12:98:98
7) Press: (X/3)4   12:110:110

Day 58—Tuesday (48 repetitions)
1) Power Snatch: 60%/1, 65%/1, 70%/1, 75%/1, 80%/1, (70%/3)3   14:14:124
2) Power Clean & Jerk: 60%/1+1, 65%/1+1, 70%/1+1,
      75%/1+1, 80%/1+1, (70%/3+1)3   22:36:146
3) Push Press: 60%/3, 65%/3, (70%/3)2   12:48:158

Day 60—Thursday (89 repetitions)
1) Snatch: 60%/2, 70%/2, 80%/2, (85%/2, 90%/1)3   15:15:173
2) Clean & Jerk: 60%/2+2, 70%/2+2, 80%/2+2, (85%/2+1, 90%/1+1)3 27:42:200
3) Clean Extension: 90%/3, 95%/3, (100%/2)2   10:52:210
4) Back Squat: 60%/3, 70%/3, 80%/3, 85%/3, 90%/2, 95%/1, (80%/3)3 24:76:234
5) Press: (X/3)4   12:88:246

Day 62—Saturday (70 repetitions)
1) Power Snatch: 60%/2, 65%/2, 70%/2, 75%/2, 80%/1,   09:09:255
2) Power Clean & Power Jerk: 60%/2+1, 65%/2+1, 70%/2+1,
    75%/2+1, 80%/1+1   14:23:269
3) Snatch Extension: (95%/2)4   08:31:277
4) Back Squat: 60%/3, 70%/3, 80%/3, 85%/3, 90%/1, 95%/1,
    80%/3, 85%/2, 90%/1   20:51:297
5) Romanian Deadlift: (90%/5)4   20:71:318

Week 10 (Pre-competition mesocycle) 254 repetitions

Day 64—Monday (89 repetitions)
1) Snatch: singles to max, (max-10, max-5, max)3   15:15:15
2) Clean & Jerk: singles to max, (max-10, max-5, max)3   30:45:45
3) Snatch High Pull: (100%/3)4   12:57:57
4) Front Squat: singles to max, (max-10, max-5, max)3   15:72:72
5) Press: (X/3)5   15:87:87

Day 65—Tuesday (38 repetitions)
1) Power Snatch: singles to max, (max-10, max-5, max)3   13:13:100
2) Power Clean & Jerk: singles to max, (max-10, max-5, max)3   26:39:126

Day 67—Thursday (71 repetitions)
1) Snatch: singles to max, (85%/2)4   14:14:140
2) Clean & Jerk: singles to max, (85%/2+1)4   24:38:164
3) Clean Extensions: (100%/2)5   10:48:174
4) Front Squat: 60%/2, 70%/2, 80%/2, 85%/2, 90%/2, 95%/1, (85%/2)2   15:63:189
5) Push Press: 60%/2, 65%/2, (70%/2)2   8:71:197

Day 69—Saturday (56 repetitions)
1) Power Snatch: 60%/2, 65%/2, (70%/2)2, (75%/2)2   12:12:209
2) Power Clean & Power Jerk: 60%/2+2, 65%/2+2,
    (70%/2+2)2, (75%/2+2)2   24:36:233
3) Back Squat: 60%/3, 70%/3, 80%/2, 85%/2, 90%/1, 95%/1,
    80%/2, 85%/2, 90%/1, 80%/3   20:56:253

Week 11 (Pre-competition mesocycle) 200 repetitions

Day 71—Monday (84 repetitions)
1) Snatch: singles to max, (max-10, max-5, max)3   15:15:15
2) Clean & Jerk: singles to max, (max-10, max-5, max)3   30:45:45
3) Snatch Extensions: (105%/3)4   12:57:57
4) Front Squat: singles to max, (max-10, max-5, max)3   15:72:72
5) Press: (X/3)4   12:84:84

Day 73—Wednesday (64 repetitions)
1) Power Snatch: singles to max, (max-10, max-5, max)3   13:13:97
2) Power Clean & Jerk: singles to max, (max-10, max-5, max)3   26:39:123
3) Back Squat: 60%/2, 70%/2, 80%/2, 90%/2, 95%/1,
      80%/3, 85%/2, 90%/1   15:54:138
4) Clean Extensions: (100%/2)5   10:64:148

Day 75—Friday (52 repetitions)
1) Snatch: 60%/1, 70%/1, 80%/1, 85%/1, 90%/1, 95%/1, 95%+/1   07:07:155
2) Clean & Jerk: 60%/1+1, 70%/1+1, 80%/1+1, 85%/1+1,
      90%/1+1, 95%/1+1, 95%+/1+1   14:21:169
3) Snatch Extensions: (105%/2)4   08:29:177
4) Front Squat: 60%/2, 70%/2, 80%/2, 85%/2, 90%/2, 95%/2,
      90%/2, 95%/1   15:44:192
5) Push Press: 60%/2, 65%/, 70%/2, 75%/2   08:52:200

Week 12 (Pre-competition Mesocycle) 136 repetitions

Day 78—Monday (57 repetitions)
1) Snatch: 60%/2, 70%/2, 80%/2, 85%/2, 90%/1   09:09:09
2) Clean & Jerk: 60%/2+1, 70%/2+1, 80%/2+1, 85%/2+1, 90%/1+1   14:23:23
3) Front Squat: 60%/2, 70%/2, 80%/2, 85%/2, 90%/1   09:32:32
4) Snatch Extension: (90%/2)4   08:40:40
5) Power Jerk: 60%/2, 65%/2, (70%/2)2, (75%/2)2   12:52:52

Day 79—Tuesday (44 repetitions)
1) Power Snatch: 60%/2, 65%/2, (70%/2)2   08:08:60
2) Power Clean & Jerk: 60%/2+2, 65%/2+2, (70%/2+2)2   16:24:76
3) Back Squat: 60%/3, 70%/3, 80%/2, (85%/2)2   12:36:88
4) Clean Extension: (85%/2)4   08:44:96

Day 81—Thursday (35 repetitions)
1) Power Snatch: 60%/2, 65%/2, 70%/2, 60%/2, 65%/2   10:10:106
2) Power Clean & Jerk: 60%/2+1, 65%/2+1, 70%/2+1,
      60%/2+1, 65%/2+1   15:25:121
3) Jumping Back Squat: (50%/2)4   08:33:129

Day 82—Friday
Rest

Day 83—Saturday
Competition

CHAPTER 12
CANDIDATE FOR MASTER OF SPORT TRAINING

A Candidate for Master of Sport (CMS) athlete is moving toward either being a lifestyler or paraprofessional. The training demands coupled with the necessity for restoration time and feeding create a situation that makes full time employment either impossible or overly demanding. A CMS lifter is often qualified for national level competition, and is adroit at performing on the competition platform. He or she may have already qualified for a minor level international competition especially at the junior level, and is sophisticated in the skills of traveling to a national competition. CMS is considered the last classification before entering the high mastery stage.

Male weightlifters who have achieved the totals in Table 12.1 are considered Candidates for Master of Sport. Female weightlifters who have achieved the totals in Table 12.2 are considered Candidates for Master of Sport.

Weight Class (kg)	56	62	69	77	85	94	105	+105
Total (kg)	175	195	220	240	255	265	275	280

Table 12.1 Candidate for Master of Sport Men Qualification

Weight Class (kg)	48	53	58	63	69	75	+75
Total (kg)	110	120	130	140	150	155	160

Table 12.2 Candidate for Master of Sport Women Qualification

CMS weightlifters should have no technical faults, display excellent speed characteristics, and have developed the capacities to train rigorously on a daily basis.

The talent level will be reflected in the speed characteristics during the preparation cycles. When lesser athletes will show significant loss of speed of movement during this phase, the talented athlete will have a much lesser drop off of speed qualities.

Exercise Selection

The exercises to be employed are smaller in number than they were for Class 1, but only to a very limited degree. They are more geared toward developing strength in an individual who has been trained to be balanced for the execution of the snatch and clean & jerk.

There will be fewer pulling movements performed from the various hang heights and from blocks. There will be no partial movements. The proportion of the various exercises will vary considerably between the preparation mesocycles and the pre-competition mesocycles.

The loading will be the primary variant rather than the exercise choices. Some of these exercises will be employed only in the event of a need for remediation, and then will be discontinued once the weakness is brought into balance.

The 18 Most Appropriate Exercises To Be Included In the Training Program of a Candidate for Master of Sport Lifter:

1) Snatch
2) Clean & Jerk
3) Cleans
4) Jerk off Rack
5) Power Snatch
6) Power Clean
7) Power Jerk
8) Snatch Pull (or Extension)
9) Clean Pull (or Extension)
10) Snatch Deadlift (Halting, Slow and Eccentric)
11) Clean Deadlift (Halting, Slow and Eccentric)
12) Romanian Deadlift (May be on blocks)
13) Back Squat (Halting, Slow and Eccentric)
14) Front Squat (Halting, Slow and Eccentric)
15) Push Press
16) Press
17) Good Mornings
18) Overhead Squat

Yearly Loading Parameters

Again, it is important to keep in mind that the figures presented are indicative of trends and approaches to program design. They may be adjusted for individual circumstances. This is the reason for the representation of ranges, which allow for specific adjustments.

The annual volume for a CMS athlete can range from 13,000 to 17,000 reps. The number of repetitions in the 90 to 100% zone for snatch and clean & jerk exercises ranges from 300 to 500.

The 90% to 100% range for snatch and clean & jerk exercises must be considered in light of the lower potential for power snatches, power cleans and power jerks. As a working percentage, if we consider a 100% power snatch to be approximately equal to an 80% classic snatch, then most of the working reps in the power snatch will fall within the 65% to 70% range of the classic snatch. A 90% power snatch would then lie at approximately 72% of the classic snatch. If we consider the percentages as absolute ranges, this inclusion of power snatches, power cleans and power jerks as snatch and clean & jerk exercises will affect both the average intensity and the intensity profiles of the training volumes.

The relative intensity in the snatch and clean & jerk exercises remains in the 73% to 75% range. The percentage of snatch lift repetitions is approximately 21% while the percentage of clean & jerk lifts is approximately 17%. This is the first class in which the number of snatch lifts exceeds the number of clean & jerk lifts. Again snatch lifts and clean & jerk lifts refer to complete lifts, i.e. classic lifts, power snatches, power cleans, power jerks.

The average volume for a four-week preparation mesocycle is 1,680, and for a four-week pre-competition mesocycle 1,072.

Loading in Zones of Intensity: Distribution of Year Volume

The percentages in Table 12.3 represent the percentage of the annual repetitions for the exercise group designated in the first column. Of course, these figures represent quantities as recorded for successful training of qualified weightlifters. Situational specifics may need to prevail as determined by the judgment of the coach.

Intensity	50-55%	60-65%	70-75%	80-85%	90-95%	100-105%	110%	Yearly Average
Snatch		10%	61%	25%	4%			72%
Clean & Jerk		9%	53%	33%	5%			74%
Snatch Pulls				31%	32%	31%	6%	91%
Clean Pulls			23%	36%	23%	13%	5%	84%
Squats	22%	28%	25%	22%	3%			68%
Fundamental Exercises	4%	13%	39%	25%	10%	8%	1%	79%

Table 12.3 Candidate for Master of Sport Zones of Intensity

Again the snatch category includes power snatches. The Clean & Jerk Category includes Power Cleans and Power Jerks. Squats includes both Front and Back Squats. Fundamental Exercises include all movements from groups 1—10 in Chapter 8 with the exclusion of presses and good mornings. The reason to exclude presses and good mornings from the calculation is the variability of the maxima of these exercises in their relationship to the maxima of the classic lifts or squats.

Calculations

A workable number of four-week preparation mesocycles is two, followed by one four-week pre-competition mesocycle as constituents of a typical macrocycle. A transitional week may follow each of the two most important competitions of the year.

The percentages of reps given over to the four weeks of the mesocycle are 30%, 27%, 23%, and 20% though not necessarily in the same order. Of course a variant of 2—3% is acceptable. (Table 12.4 and Graph 12.1)

Prep Month 1	Week 1	Week 2	Week 3	Week 4
Volume	504	386	453	336
Prep Month 2	Week 5	Week 6	Week 7	Week 8
Volume	504	453	386	336
Pre-Competition	Week 9	Week 10	Week 11	Week 12
Volume	321	289	247	214

Table 12.4 Candidate for Master of Sport Weekly Volume

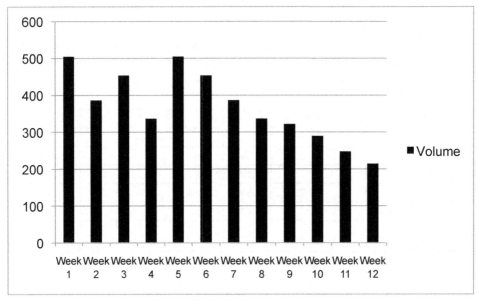

Graph 12.1 CMS weekly volume.

Week	1	2	3	4	5	6	7	8	9	10	11	12
Training Days	5-6	5	5	4	5-6	5	5	4	4	4	4	3

Table 12.5 Candidate for Master of Sport Training Days per Week

The daily volumes can then be calculated using the weekly volumes and the daily percentages. The preparation mesocycles are highlighted in gray. (Table 12.6 and Graph 12.2)

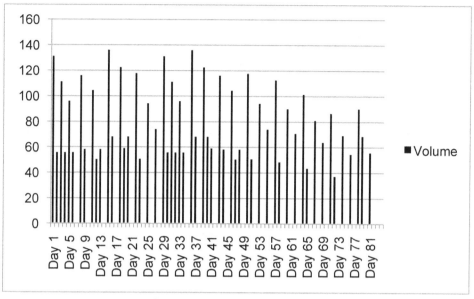

Graph 12.2 CMS Daily Volumes

Table 12.6 Candidate for Master of Sport Daily Volume

Week	Day	Week Vol	Daily %	Day Vol
Week 1	Day 1	504	26%	131
	Day 2		11%	55
	Day 3		22%	111
	Day 4		11%	55
	Day 5		19%	96
	Day 6		11%	55
	Day 7		0%	0
Week 2	Day 8	386	30%	116
	Day 9		15%	58
	Day 10		0%	0
	Day 11		27%	104
	Day 12		13%	50
	Day 13		15%	58
	Day 14		0%	0

Week 3	Day 15	453	30%	136
	Day 16		15%	68
	Day 17		0%	0
	Day 18		27%	122
	Day 19		13%	59
	Day 20		15%	68
	Day 21		0%	0
Week 4	Day 22	336	35%	118
	Day 23		15%	50
	Day 24		0%	0
	Day 25		28%	94
	Day 26		0%	0
	Day 27		22%	74
	Day 28		0%	0
Week 5	Day 29	504	26%	131
	Day 30		11%	55
	Day 31		22%	111
	Day 32		11%	55
	Day 33		19%	96
	Day 34		11%	55
	Day 35		0%	0
Week 6	Day 36	453	30%	136
	Day 37		15%	68
	Day 38		0%	0
	Day 39		27%	122
	Day 40		15%	68
	Day 41		13%	59
	Day 42		0%	0
Week 7	Day 43	386	30%	116
	Day 44		15%	58
	Day 45		0%	0
	Day 46		27%	104
	Day 47		13%	50
	Day 48		15%	58
	Day 49		0%	0

WEIGHTLIFTING PROGRAMMING

Week 8	Day 50	336	35%	118
	Day 51		15%	50
	Day 52		0%	0
	Day 53		28%	94
	Day 54		0%	0
	Day 55		22%	74
	Day 56		0%	0
Week 9	Day 57	321	35%	112
	Day 58		15%	48
	Day 59		0%	0
	Day 60		28%	90
	Day 61		0%	0
	Day 62		22%	71
	Day 63		0%	0
Week 10	Day 64	289	35%	101
	Day 65		15%	43
	Day 66		0%	0
	Day 67		28%	81
	Day 68		0%	0
	Day 69		22%	64
	Day 70		0%	0
Week 11	Day 71	247	35%	86
	Day 72		15%	37
	Day 73		0%	0
	Day 74		28%	69
	Day 75		0%	0
	Day 76		22%	54
	Day 77		0%	0
Week 12	Day 78	214	42%	90
	Day 79		32%	68
	Day 80		0%	0
	Day 81		26%	56
	Day 82		0%	0
	Day 83		0%	0
	Day 84		0%	0

SAMPLE CANDIDATE FOR MASTER OF SPORT TRAINING PROGRAM

The numbers to the right represent respectively the number of repetitions in the exercise, the number of repetitions in the workout and the running cumulative number of repetitions for the week.

Week 1 (Preparation Mesocycle) 504 repetitions

Day 1—Monday (131 repetitions)
1) Back Squat: 60%/4, 70%/4, (75%/4)3   20:20:20
2) Snatch: 60%/4, 70%/4, (75%/4)3   20:40:40
3) Clean & Jerk: 60%/4+1, 70%/4+1, (75%/4+1)3   25:65:65
4) Jerk off Rack: 70%/4, (80%/3)3   13:78:78
5) Clean Extension: (85%/4)5   20:98:98
6) Snatch Deadlift: (105%/4)4   16:114:114
7) Press: (X/4)4   16:130:130

Day 2—Tuesday (55 repetitions)
1) Power Snatch: 60%/3, 65%/3, (70%/3)3   15:15:145
2) Power Clean & Power Jerk: 60%/3+2, 65%/3+2, (70%/3+2)2   20:35:165
3) Snatch Extension: (90%/4)4   16:41:181
4) Push Press: 60%/3, 65%/3, (70%/3)3   15:56:196

Day 3—Wednesday (111 repetitions)
1) Back Squat: 60%/3, 70%/3, (80%/3)2   12:12:208
2) Snatch: 60%/3, 70%/3, (80%/3)2   12:24:220
3) Clean & Jerk: 60%/3+1, 70%/3+1, (80%/3+1)2   16:40:236
4) Behind the Neck Push Press: 60%/4, 65%/4, (70%/3)3   17:57:253
5) Clean High Pull off blocks: (85%/4)4   16:73:269
6) Snatch Deadlift on blocks: (85%/4)4   16:89:285
7) Good Morning: (X/6)4   24:113:309

Day 4—Thursday (55 repetitions)
1) Power Snatch & Overhead Squat: 60%/3+3, 65%/3+3, (70%/3+3)2   24:24:333
2) Power Clean & Power Jerk: 60%/3+3, 65%/3+3, (70%/3+3)2   24:48:357
3) Press: (X/2)4   08:56:365

Day 5—Friday (96 repetitions)
1) Front Squat: 60%/4, 70%/4, (75%/4)3   20:20:385
2) Snatch: 60%/4, 70%/4, (75%/4)2   16:36:401
3) Clean & Jerk: 60%/4+1, 70%/4+1, (75%/4+1)2   20:46:421
4) Snatch High Pull: (90%/4)5   20:66:441
5) Romanian Deadlift: (85%/5)4   20:86:461
6) Jerk Drive: (80%/3)4   12:98:473

Day 6—Saturday (55 repetitions)
1) Power Snatch: 60%/2, 65%/2, (70%/2)3   10:10:483
2) Power Clean & Jerk: 60%/2+2, 65%/2+2, (70%/2+2)3   20:30:503

Week 2 (Preparation Mesocycle) 386 repetitions

Day 8—Monday (116 repetitions)
1) Back Squat: 60%/4, 70%/4, (80%/4)2   16:16:16
2) Snatch: 60%/4, 70%/4, (80%/4)2   16:32:32
3) Clean & Jerk: 60%/4+1, 70%/4+1, (80%/4+1)2   20:52:52
4) Jerk off Rack: 70%/3, (80%/3)3   12:64:64
5) Snatch High Pull: (90%/4)4   16:80:80
6) Romanian Deadlift: (90%/5)4   20:100:100
7) Press: (X/3)4   12:112:112

Day 9—Tuesday (58 repetitions)
1) Power Snatch: 60%/3, 65%/3, (70%/3)3   15:15:127
2) Power Clean & Power Jerk: 60%/3+2, 65%/3+2, (70%/3+2)3   25:40:152
3) Clean Extension: 80%/4, (85%/4)4   20:60:172

Day 10—Wednesday
Day Off

Day 11—Thursday (104 repetitions)
1) Front Squat: 60%/4, 70%/4, (80%/4)2   16:16:188
2) Snatch: 60%/4, 70%/4, (80%/4)3   20:36:208
3) Clean: 60%/4, 70%/4, (80%/4)3   20:56:228
4) Jerk off Rack: 60%/4, 70%/4, (80%/4)2   16:72:244
5) Snatch Extension: (95%/4)4   16:88:260
6) Good Morning: (X/5)4   20:108:280

Day 12—Friday (50 repetitions)
1) Power Snatch & Overhead Squat: 60%/3+3, 65%/3+3, (70%/3+3)3   30:30:310
2) Power Clean & Power Jerk: 60%/3+3, 65%/3+3, (70%/3+3)2   24:54:334

Day 13—Saturday (58 repetitions)
1) Back Squat: 60%/3, 70%/3, (80%/3)3   15:15:349
2) Snatch: 60%/3, 70%/3, (80%/2)2   10:25:359
3) Clean & Jerk: 60%/3+1, 70%/3+1, (80%/2+1)2   14:39:373
4) Clean Extension: (85%/4)4   16:55:389

Week 3 (Preparation Mesocycle) 453 repetitions

Day 15—Monday (136 repetitions)
1) Back Squat: 60%/4, 70%/4, (80%/4)4   24:24:24
2) Snatch: 60%/4, 70%/4, (80%/4)3   20:44:44
3) Clean & Jerk: 60%/4+1, 70%/4+1, (80%/4+1)3   25:69:69
4) Clean High Pull: (85%/4)5   20:89:89
5) Behind the Neck Power Jerk: 60%/4, 65%/4, (70%/4)3   20:109:109
6) Good Morning: (X/6)4   24:133:133

Day 16—Tuesday (68 repetitions)
1) Power Snatch & Overhead Squat: 60%/3+3, 65%/3+3, (70%/3+3)3   30:30:163
2) Power Clean & Power Jerk: 60%/3+3, 65%/3+3, (70%/3+3)3   30:60:193
3) Press: (X/3)4   12:72:205

Day 17—Wednesday
Rest

Day 18—Thursday (122 repetitions)
1) Front Squat: 60%/4, 70%/4, (80%/4)3   20:20:225
2) Snatch: 60%/3, 70%/3, (80%/3)3   15:35:240
3) Clean: 60%/3, 70%/3, (80%/3)3   15:50:255
4) Jerk off Rack: 60%/4, 70%/4, (80%/4)3   20:70:275
5) Snatch High Pull: (95%/4)5   20:90:295
6) Push Press: 60%/4, 65%/4, (70%/4)3   20:110:315
7) Press: (X/3)4   12:122:327

Day 19—Friday (59 repetitions)
1) Power Snatch: 60%/2, 65%/2, (70%/2)3   10:10:337
2) Power Clean & Jerk: 60%/2+2, 65%/2+2, (70%/2+2)3   20:30:357
3) Romanian Deadlift: (90%/5)5   25:55:382

Day 20—Saturday (68 repetitions)
1) Back Squat: 60%/3, 70%/3, 80%/3, 85%/2, (80%/3)2   17:17:399
2) Snatch: 60%/2, 70%/2, 80%/2, (85%/2)2   10:27:409
3) Clean: 60%/2, 70%/, 80%/2, (85%/2)2   10:37:419
4) Clean Extension: (85%/5)4   20:57:439
5) Press: (X/4)4   16:73:455

Week 4 (Preparation mesocycle) 336 repetitions

Day 22—Monday (118 repetitions)
1) Back Squat: 60%/4, 70%/4, (80%/4)4   24:24:24
2) Snatch: 60%/4, 70%/4, (80%/4)4   24:48:48
3) Clean: 60%/4, 70%/4, (80%/4)3   20:68:68
4) Jerk off Rack: 60%/4, 70%/4, (80%/4)4   24:92:92
5) Push Press: 60%/4, 65%/4, (70%/4)3   20:112:112

Day 23—Tuesday (50 repetitions)
1) Power Snatch & Behind the Neck Push Press & Overhead Squat:
    60%/2+2+2, 65%/2+2+2, (70%/2+2+2)2   24:24:136
2) Power Clean & Front Squat & Power Jerk:
    60%/2+2+2, 65%/2+2+2, (70%/2+2+2)2   24:48:160

Day 24—Wednesday
Rest

Day 25—Thursday (94 repetitions)
1) Front Squat: 60%/4, 70%/4, (80%/4)4   24:24:184
2) Snatch: 60%/3, 70%/3, (80%/3)3   15:39:199
3) Clean & Jerk: 60%/3+2, 70%/3+2, (80%/3+1)3   22:61:221
4) Clean Extensions: (90%/4)4   16:77:237
5) Snatch Deadlift: (105%/3)4   12:89:249
6) Press: (X/3)4   12:101:261

Day 26—Friday
Rest

Day 27—Saturday (74 repetitions)
1) Back Squat: 60%/3, 70%/3, (80%/3)4   18:18:279
2) Snatch: 60%/2, 70%/2, 80%/2, 85%/2   08:26:287
3) Clean & Jerk: 60%/2+1, 70%/2+1, 80%/2+1, 85%/2+1   12:38:299
4) Snatch High Pull: (95%/4)5   20:58:319
5) Push Press: 60%/3, 65%/3, (70%/3)3   15:73:334

Week 5 (Preparation Mesocycle) 504 repetitions

Day 29—Monday (131 repetitions)
1) Back Squat: 60%/4, 70%/4, 80%/4, 85%/3, (80%/4)2   23:23:23
2) Snatch: 60%/4, 70%/3, (80%/4)4   24:47:47
3) Clean & Jerk: 60%/4+1, 70%/4+1, (80%4+1)4   30:77:77
4) Snatch Extension: (95%/4)5   20:97:97
5) Romanian Deadlift: (90%/5)4   20:117:117
6) Power Jerk: 60%/3, (70%/3)3   12:129:129

Day 30—Tuesday (55 repetitions)
1) Power Snatch: 60%/4, 65%/4, (70%/4)3   20:20:149
2) Power Clean & Power Jerk: 60%/4+2, 65%/4+2, (70%/4+2)3   30:50:179
3) Press; (X/3)4   12:62:191

Day 31—Wednesday (111 repetitions)
1) Front Squat: 60%/4, 70%/4, (80%/4)4   24:24:215
2) Snatch High Pull & Snatch: 60%/3+1, 70%/3+1, (80%/3+1)3   20:44:235
3) Clean High Pull & Clean: 60%/3+1, 70%/3+1, (80%/3+1)3   20:64:255
4) Clean Extensions: (90%/4)5   20:84:275
5) Jerk off Rack: 60%/4, 70%/4, (80%/4)3   20:104:295

Day 32—Thursday (55 repetitions)
1) Snatch: 60%/2, 70%/2, 80%/2, 85%/2   08:08:303
2) Clean & Jerk: 60%/2+2, 70%/2+2, 80%/2+2, 85%/2+1   15:23:318
3) Snatch High Pull: (95%/3)4   12:35:330
4) Push Press: 60%/3, 65%/3, (70%/3)4   18:53:348

Day 33—Friday (96 repetitions)
1) Power Snatch & Behind the Neck Push Press & Overhead Squat:
    60%/3+3+3, 65%/3+3+3, (70%/3+3+3)3   45:45:393
2) Power Clean & Front Squat & Power Jerk:
    60%/3+3+3, 65%/3+3+3, (70%/3+3+3)3   45:90:438
3) Clean Deadlift: (105%/2)4   08:98:446

Day 34—Saturday (55 repetitions)
1) Back Squat: 60%/3, 70%/3, 80%/3, 85%/3, 90%/1   13:13:459
2) Power Snatch: 60%/3, 65%/3, 70%/3, 75%/1, 70%/3, 75%/1, 70%/2   16:29:475
3) Power Clean & Power Jerk: 60%/3+1, 65%/3+1,
    70%/3+1, 75%/1+1, 70%/3+1, 75%/1+1, 70%/2+1   23:52:498
4) Press: (X/2)4   08:60:506

Week 6 (Preparation Mesocycle) 453 repetitions

Day 36—Monday (136 repetitions)
1) Back Squat: 60%/4, 70%/4, (80%/4, 85%/2)3   26:26:26
2) Snatch: 60%/4, 70%/4, (80%/4, 85%/2)3   26:52:52
3) Clean: 60%/4, 70%/4, (80%/4, 85%/2)3   26:78:78
4) Snatch High Pull: (95%/4)5   20:98:98
5) Clean Deadlift: (105%/3)4   12:110:110
6) Good Morning: (X/6)4   24:134:134

Day 37—Tuesday (68 repetitions)
1) Power Snatch: 60%/4, 65%/4, (70%/4, 75%/1)3   23:23:157
2) Power Clean & Power Jerk: 60%/4+2, 65%/4+2,
    (70%/4+1, 75%/1+1)3   33:56:190
3) Snatch Deadlift: (105%/3)4   12:68:202

Day 38--Wednesday
Rest

Day 39—Thursday (122 repetitions)
1) Front Squat: 60%/4, 70%/4, (80%/4, 85%/2)3   26:26:228
2) Snatch: 60%/3, 70%/3, 80%/3, (85%/3)3   18:44:246
3) Clean & Jerk: 60%/3+1, 70%/3+1, 80%/3+1, (85%/3+1)3   24:68:270
4) Jerk off Rack: (80%/4)2, (85%/3)2   14:82:284
5) Clean High Pull: (90%/4)5   20:102:304
6) Good Morning; (X/5)4   20:122:324

Day 40—Friday (68 repetitions)
1) Power Snatch & Overhead Squat: 60%/3+3, 65%/3+3, (70%/3+3)3   30:30:354
2) Power Clean & Power Jerk: 60%/3+3, 65%/3+3, (70%/3+3)3   30:60:384
3) Press: (X/2)4   08:68:392

Day 41—Saturday (55 repetitions)
1) Back Squat: 60%/2, 70%/2, 80%/2, 85%/2, 90%/1, 85%/2   11:11:403
2) Snatch: 60%/2, 70%/2, 80%/2, 85%/2, 90%/1, 85%/2   11:22:414
3) Clean & Jerk: 60%/2+1, 70%/2+1, 80%/2+1, 85%/2+1,
      90%/1+1, 85%/2+1   17:39:431
4) Snatch High Pull: (100%/4)5   20:59:451

Week 7 (preparation Mesocycle) 386 repetitions

Day 43—Monday (116 repetitions)
1) Back Squat: 60%/3, 70%/3, 80%/3, (85%/3)3   18:18:18
2) Snatch: 60%/3, 70%/3, 80%/3, (85%/3)3   18:36:36
3) Clean & Jerk: 60%/3+1, 70%/3+1, 80%/3+1, (85%/3+1)3   24:60:60
4) Jerk: 80%/3, (85%/3)3   12:72:72
5) Clean High Pull: (90%/3)5   15:87:87
6) Good Morning: (X/5)4   20:117:117

Day 44—Tuesday (58 repetitions)
1) Power Snatch: 60%/2, 65%/2, (70%/2)3   10:10:127
2) Power Clean & Power Jerk: 60%/2+2, 65%/2+2, (70%/2+2)3   20:30:147
3) Snatch Extensions: (95%/3)5   15:45:162
4) Press: (X/3)4   12:57:174

Day 45—Wednesday
Rest

Day 46—Thursday (104 repetitions)
1) Front Squat: 60%/4, 70%/4, (80%/4)5   28:28:202
2) Snatch: 60%/3, 70%/3, 80%/3, (85%/3)3   18:44:220
3) Clean & Jerk: 60%/3+1, 70%/3+1, 80%/3+1, (85%/3+1)3   24:68:244
4) Clean Extensions: (90%/4)5   20:88:264
5) Good Morning: (X/5)4   20:108:284

Day 47—Friday (50 repetitions)
1) Power Snatch & Overhead Squat: 60%/2+3, 65%/2+3, (70%/2+3)3   25:25:309

Day 49—Saturday (58 repetitions)
1) Back Squat: 60%/2, 70%/2, 80%/2, 85%/2, 90%/2, 85%/2, 90%/1   13:13:13
2) Snatch: 60%/2, 70%/2, 80%/2, (85%/2, 90%/1)2   12:25:25
3) Clean & Jerk: 60%/2+1, 70%/2+1, 80%/2+1, (85%/2+1, 90%/1+1)2   19:44:44
4) Press: (X/3)4   12:56:56

Week 8 (Preparation Mesocycle) 336 repetitions

Day 50—Monday (118 repetitions)
1) Back Squat: 60%/4, 70%/4, (80%/4, 85%/3)3   29:29:29
2) Snatch: 60%/4, 70%/4, (80%/4, 85%/3)3   29:58:58
3) Clean & Jerk: 60%/4+1, 70%/4+1, (80%/4+1, 85%/3+1)3   37:95:95
4) Snatch High Pull: (100%/4)5   20:115:115

Day 51—Tuesday (50 repetitions)
1) Power Snatch: 60%/1, 65%/1, 70%/1, (75%/1)3, (70%/3)3   15:15:130
2) Power Clean & Jerk: 60%/1+1, 65%/1+1, 70%/1+1,
       (75%/1+1)3, (70%/3+1)3   24:39:154
3) Jerk: 70%/3, 80%/3, (85%/3)2   12:51:166

Day 52—Wednesday
Rest

Day 53—Thursday (94 repetitions)
1) Front Squat: 60%/4, 70%/4, (80%/4, 85%/3)3   29:29:195
2) Snatch: 60%/2, 70%/2, 80%/2, (85%/2, 90%/1)3   15:44:210
3) Clean & Jerk: 60%/2+1, 70%/2+1, 80%/2+1, (85%/2+1, 90%/1+1)3   24:68:234
4) Snatch Extension: (105%/3)5   15:83:249
5) Romanian Deadlift: (90%/4)4   16:99:265

Day 54—Friday
Rest

Day 55—Saturday (74 repetitions)
1) Back Squat: 60%/3, 70%/3, 80%/3, 85%/3, 90%/2, 85%/2, 90%/1   17:17:282
2) Power Snatch: 60%/2, 65%/2, 70%/2, 75%/2, 80%/1, 70%/2, 75%/1   12:29:294
3) Power Clean & Power Jerk: 60%/2+1, 65%/2+1, 70%/2+1,
       75%/2+1, 80%/1+1, 70%/2+1, 75%/1+1   19:48:313
4) Jerk: 70%/3, 80%/3, (85%/3)3   15:63:328
5) Press: (X/3)4   12:75:340

Week 9 (Pre-competition Macrocycle) 321 repetitions

Day 57—Monday (112 repetitions)
1) Snatch: 60%/1, 70%/1, 80%/1, 85%/1, 90%/1, 95%/1, (80%/3)3   15:15:15
2) Clean & Jerk: 60%/1+1, 70%/1+1, 80%/1+1, 85%/1+1,
       90%/1+1, 95%/1+1, (80%/3+1)3   24:39:39
3) Snatch High Pull: 95%/3, (100%/3)2, (105%/3)2   15:54:54
4) Front Squat: 60%/3, 70%/3, 80%/3, (85%/3)4   21:75:75
5) Power Jerk: 60%/3, 65%/3, 70%/3, 75%/3, 70%/3, 75%/2, 70%/3   20:95:95
6) Good Morning: (X/5)4   20:115:115

Day 58—Tuesday (48 repetitions)
1) Power Snatch: 60%/1, 65%/1, 70%/1, (75%/1)3, (70%/3)3   15:15:130
2) Power Clean & Power Jerk: 60%/1+1, 65%/1+1,
        70%/1+1, (75%/1+1)3, (70%/3+1)3   24:39:154
3) Clean Extension: 85%/2, 95%/2, (100%/2)3   10:49:164

Day 59—Wednesday
Rest

Day 60—Thursday (90 repetitions)
1) Snatch: 60%/2, 70%/2, 80%/2, (85%/2, 90%/1)3   15:15:179
2) Clean & Jerk: 60%/2+1, 70%/2+1, 80%/2+1, (85%/2+1, 90%/1+1)3   24:39:203
3) Snatch Extension: (105%/3)5   15:54:218
4) Back Squat: 60%/2, 70%/2, 80%/2, 85%/2, (90%/2)4   16:70:234
5) Press: (X/4)4   16:86:250

Day 61—Friday
Rest

Day 62—Saturday (71 repetitions)
1) Power Snatch & Overhead Squat: 60%/2+2, 65%/2+2,
        (70%/2+2)2, (75%/2+2)2   24:24:274
2) Power Clean & Power Jerk: 60%/2+2, 65%/2+2,
        (70%/2+2)2, (75%/2+2)2   24:48:298
3) Clean Extension: 85%/2, 95%/2, (105%/2)3   10:58:308
4) Front Squat: 60%/2, 70%/2, 80%/2, 85%/2 (90%/2)2   12:70:320

Week 10 (Pre-Competition Mesocycle) 289 repetitions

Day 64—Monday (101 repetitions)
1) Snatch: singles to max, (max-10, max-5, max)3   15:15:15
2) Clean & Jerk: singles to max, (max-10, max-5, max)3   30:45:45
3) Clean Extension: (105%/2)5   10:55:55
4) Front Squat: singles to max, (max-10, max-5, max03   15:70:70
5) Jerk: 70%/2, 80%/2, (85%2)2, (90%/2)2   12:82:82
6) Good Morning: (X/5)4   20:102:102

Day 65—Tuesday (43 repetitions)
1) Power Snatch: singles to max, (max-10, max-5, max)3   12:12:114
2) Power Clean & Power Jerk: singles to max, (max-10, max-5, max)3   24:36:138
3) Press: (X/3)4   12:48:150

Day 66—Wednesday
Rest

Day 67—Thursday (81 repetitions)
1) Snatch: singles to max, (85%/2)4   14:14:164
2) Clean & Jerk: singles to max, (85%/2+1)4   24:38:188
3) Snatch High Pull; (105%/2)5   10:48:198
4) Back Squat: singles to max, (max-10, max-5, max)3   15:63:213
5) Push Press: 60%/3, 65%/3, (70%/3)3   15:78:228

Day 68—Friday
Rest

Day 69—Saturday (64 repetitions)
1) Power Snatch; 60%/2, 65%/2, (70%/2, 75%/1, 80%/1)2   12:12:240
2) Power Clean & Jerk: 60%/2+1, 65%/2+1,
        (70%/2+1, 75%/1+1, 80%/1+1)2   20:32:260
3) Front Squat: 60%/2, 70%/2, 80%/2, 85%/2, (90%/2)3   14:46:274
4) Clean Extension: 90%/3, (100%/3)4   15:61:289

Week 11 (Pre-competition Mesocycle) 247 repetitions

Day 71—Monday (86 repetitions)
1) Snatch: singles to max. max-10, max-5, max, (90%/2)3   12:12:12
2) Clean & Jerk: singles to max, max-10, max-5, max (90%/2+1)3   18:30:30
3) Clean High Pull: (95%/2)5   10:40:40
4) Front Squat: singles to max, max-10, max-5, max (90%/2)3   12:52:52
5) Push Press: 60%/3, 65%/3, 70%/3, 75%/2, 70%/3   14:66:66
6) Good Morning: (X/5)4   20:86:86

Day 72—Tuesday (37 repetitions)
1) Power Snatch: singles to max, max-10, max-5, max   07:07:93
2) Power Clean & Power Jerk: singles to max, max-10, max-5, max   14:21:107
3) Snatch Extension: (105%/3)5   15:36:122

Day 73—Wednesday
Rest

Day 74—Thursday (69 repetitions)
1) Snatch: 60%/2, 70%/2, 80%/2, 85%/2, 90%/2, 95%/1   11:11:133
2) Clean & Jerk: 60%/2+1, 70%/2+1, 80%/2+1, 85%/2+1,
        90%/1+1, 95%/1+1   16:27:149
3) Clean Extension: 100%/2, (105%/2)4   10:37:159
4) Back Squat: Singles to max, (max-10, max-5, max)3   15:52:174
5) Press: (X/4)4   16:68:190

Day 75—Friday
Rest

Day 76—Saturday (54 repetitions)
1) Snatch: 60%/2, 70%/2, 80%/2, (85%/2)2   12:12:202
2) Clean & Jerk: 60%/2+2, 70%/2+2, 80%/2+2, (85%/2+1)2   18:30:220
3) Snatch Extension: (105%/2)3   06:36:226
4) Front Squat: 60%/2, 70%/2, 80%/2, (85%/2)2   10:46:236
5) Press: (X/3)3   09:55:245

Week 12 (Pre-Competition Mesocycle) 214 repetitions

Day 78—Monday (90 repetitions)
1) Snatch: 60%/2, 70%/2, 80%/1, 85%/1, 90%/1, 95%/1, (85%/1)4   12:12:12
2) Clean & Jerk: 60%/2+1, 70%/2+1, 80%/2+1, 85%/1+1,
      90%/1+1, 95%/1+1, (85%/1+1)3   19:31:31
3) Snatch Extension: (95%/2)5   10:41:41
4) Front Squat: 60%/3, 70%/3, 80%/3, 85%/2, 90%/1, 80%/3, (85%/2)3   19:60:60
5) Press: (X/3)5   15:75:75

Day 79—Tuesday (68 repetitions)
1) Snatch: 60%/2, 70%/2, 80%/1, 85%/1, 90%/1, (85%/1)3   10:10:85
2) Clean & Jerk: 60%/2+1, 70%/2+1, 80%/1+1, 85%/1+1,
      90%/1+1, (85%/1+1)3   18:28:103
3) Back Squat: 60%/2, 70%/2, 80%/2, 85%/2, 90%/1, (85%/2)2   13:41:116
4) Snatch High Pull: (85%/3)4   12:53:128

Day 80—Wednesday
Rest

Day 81—Thursday (56 repetitions)
1) Power Snatch:60%/2, 65%/2, (70%/2)3   10:10:138
2) Power Clean & Power Jerk: 60%/2+2, 65%/2+2, (70%/2+2)3   20:30:158
3) Jumping Back Squat: (50%/3)4   12:42:170
4) Press: (X/2)4   08:50:178

Day 82—Friday
Rest

Day 83—Saturday
Competition

CHAPTER 13
MASTER OF SPORT

The Master of Sport Athlete is a weightlifter that is the equivalent of a full time professional. Master of Sport is considered the lowest stage of the High Mastery category. Because of the number of times training per day, the amount of time devoted to pre-workout and post-workout restoration, as well as the numerous feedings that are an absolute necessity, a Master of Sport weightlifter will not have enough time, nor energy, to work for a living. Support for these athletes in many countries is provided by the government through the national Olympic Committee. In some situations, a wealthy benefactor can provide support for a promising and talented lifter. Still in many sports in many countries, financial support comes from parents and family.

For an athlete to reach this level, he or she should regularly be placing in the top three in the weight class at national and/or continental championships. It is not uncommon for national junior and youth records to have been set by Master Athletes. Master lifters may also frequently be named to junior and youth world championships teams. They are essentially waiting to move forward and take their places as national senior champions and members of senior world national teams and Olympic teams. It should not need to be said, but athletes reaching this point have considerable talent for the sport.

Male weightlifters who have achieved the totals in Table 13.1 are considered Masters of Sport. Female weightlifters who have achieved the totals in Table 13.2 are considered Masters of Sport.

Weight Class (kg)	56	62	69	77	85	94	105	+105
Total (kg)	205	230	255	280	295	310	320	325

Table 13.1 Master of Sport Men Qualification

Weight Class (kg)	48	53	58	63	69	75	+75
Total (kg)	130	140	150	160	170	180	190

Table 13.2 Master of Sport Women Qualification

Athletes in this class should have excellent technique and speed characteristics. They should have the genetics to proceed further without significant injuries or nagging injuries that will interfere or inhibit training. It is during this stage of development that these factors will begin to insert themselves into the progression of the athletic career.

Exercise Selection

The exercises to be employed are the same as those employed for the Candidate for Master of Sport Class. They are more geared toward developing strength in an individual who has been trained to be balanced for the execution of the snatch and clean & jerk. There will be fewer pulling movements performed from the various hang heights and from blocks. There will be very few partial movements unless the athlete is recovering from an injury. The proportion of classical lifts and their derivatives to strength building exercises will vary considerably between the preparation mesocycles and the pre-competition mesocycles.

The loading will be the primary variant rather than the exercise choices. Some of these exercises will be employed only in the event of a need for remediation, and then will be discontinued once the weakness is brought into balance. Again, the variety of exercises will diminish as the competition draws near. *On blocks* means the lifter is standing on a block that places the instep very nearly touching the bar at the starting position. *Off blocks* means that the bar is resting on blocks that elevate it off the floor prior to the start of each repetition.

The 18 Most Appropriate Exercises To Be Included In the Training Program of a Master of Sport Lifter:

1) Snatch (from the hang, on blocks, off blocks)
2) Clean & Jerk
3) Cleans (from the hang, on blocks, off blocks)
4) Jerk off Rack
5) Power Snatch (from the hang, on blocks, off blocks)
6) Power Clean (from the hang, on blocks, off blocks)
7) Power Jerk
8) Snatch Pull (or Extension, on blocks, off blocks)
9) Clean Pull (or Extension, on blocks, off blocks)
10) Snatch Deadlift (Halting, Slow and Eccentric, on blocks)
11) Clean Deadlift (Halting, Slow and Eccentric, on blocks)
12) Romanian Deadlift (May be on blocks)
13) Back Squat (Halting, Slow and Eccentric)
14) Front Squat (Halting, Slow and Eccentric)
15) Push Press
16) Press (Standing, Seated or Supine)
17) Good Mornings
18) Overhead Squat

Yearly Loading Parameters

At this point it is important for the coach to realize that weightlifters that have achieved Master of Sport status are talented individuals who have demonstrated a drive and intensity that has placed them at this point in their career. They are susceptible to certain training trends that are represented by the figures in this section and yet they are each individuals with different combinations of abilities and aptitudes that must be considered in the planning of training.

The common error that often takes place with newer coaches throughout their early training experience is to try to adhere too closely to the prescribed numbers. One must keep in mind that the numbers presented are empirically derived from the training of experienced, talented weightlifters. They do not, however, cover all of the individuals that a coach might encounter, especially if he is in a professional situation. This is why it is important for younger coaches to be able to consult regularly with veteran coaches.

The annual volume for a MS (Master of Sport) weightlifter can range from 16,000 to as high as 21,000 repetitions. The number of repetitions in the 90%—100% zone for snatch and clean and jerk exercises can range from 300—600. In this calculation, the cleans and jerks are counted separately.

When determining the actual volume, the restoration capacity of the athlete must be taken into consideration. The lighter and younger the athlete, the greater the volume that can be accommodated. For talented, light, and young athletes the volume can range in the higher numbers, while for older, heavier athletes, the volume will be considerably lower.

The relative intensity in the snatch and clean & jerk exercises should be in the 73% to 77% range. Again, it is important to keep in mind that these exercises include snatches, power snatches, cleans, jerks, power cleans and power jerks. The majority of power snatch, power clean and power jerk exercises will fall in the 60% to 80% zones, and thus will have the effect of lowering the average intensity.

Master of Sport can also be further divided into two stages. There is the minimum level of attainment, and then a second stage for those who have placed from 3 to 10th place in the Republic Championships (a term referring to the old Soviet republics, which are now independent nations). Since placings are relative designations, the coach may simply wish to divide the range between Master of Sport and International Master of Sport in half to determine the cutoff between Stage 1 and Stage 2.

The average volume for a four-week preparation mesocycle for Stage 1 Masters should average 1,900 repetitions, while the four-week pre-competition mesocycle should average 1,330. Stage 2 Masters should average 2,280 for a four-week preparation mesocycle and 1,410 reptitions for a four-week pre-competition mesocycle.

The maximum number of hours per week spent in training should be in the 30 to 32 hour range.

Loading in Zones of Intensity: Distribution of Year Volume

The percentages in Table 13.3 represent the percentage of the annual volume for the exercise group designated in the first column. Remember that these are guideline numbers that have been proven to be effective. They may be modified by a skillful coach depending on the individual athlete's situation.

The snatch exercises include all snatches and power snatches. Clean & jerk exercises include all cleans, power cleans, jerks and power jerks. The Fundamental Exercises include all exercises in Groups 1—10 as listed in Chapter 8.

Intensity	50-55%	60-65%	70-75%	80-85%	90-95%	100-105%	110%	Yearly Average
Snatch		16%	63%	19%	2%			71%
Clean & Jerk		11%	55%	31%		3%		73%
Snatch Pulls				25%	37%	32%	6%	91%
Clean Pulls			20%	38%	24%	13%	5%	84%
Squats	22%	30%	25%	20%	2%			66%
Fundamental Exercises*	4%	13%	39%	25%	10%	8%	1%	79%

Table 13.3 Master of Sport Zones of Intensity
Does not include good mornings or presses

Calculations

For Master Athletes it is advisable to schedule the major peak after three four-week preparation mesocycles followed by a four-week pre-competition mesocycle. This means that the weekly volumes must be varied during the preparation phase so that they do fall into a regular pattern and can build to a high volume point that sufficiently taxes the endocrines. The percentage of the 1,900 repetitions of the preparation mesocycle and the 1,330 repetitions of the pre-competition mesocycle given over to the four weeks are 30%, 27%, 23%, and 20% in any order. (Table 13.4)

A 17th tapering week should precede the competition. The volume should be approximately 150 repetitions. This is therefore a 17-week cycle. The data from Table 13.4 is represented in Graph 13.1.

Prep Month 1	Week 1	Week 2	Week 3	Week 4
Volume	570	380	513	437
Prep Month 2	Week 5	Week 6	Week 7	Week 8
Volume	570	513	380	437
Prep Month 3	Week 9	Week 10	Week 11	Week 12
Volume	570	437	513	380
Pre-Comp Month	Week 13	Week 14	Week 15	Week 16
Volume	399	359	305	266

Table 13.4 Master of Sport Weekly Volume

Week	1	2	3	4	5	6	7	8	9	10	11	12	13	14	15	16	17
Training Days	6	4	6	5	6	6	4	5	6	5	6	4	5	4	4	4	3

Table 13.5 Master of Sport Training Days per Week

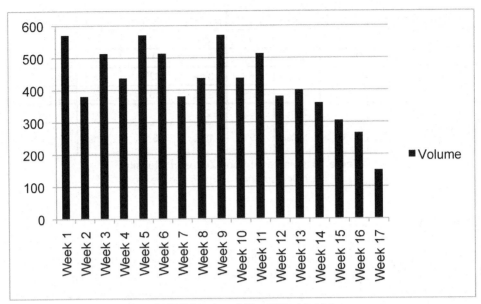

Graph 13.1 Master of Sport Weekly Volume

The daily volumes can then be calculated using the weekly volumes and the daily percentages. The preparation mesocycles are highlighted in gray. (Table 13.6 and Graph 13.2)

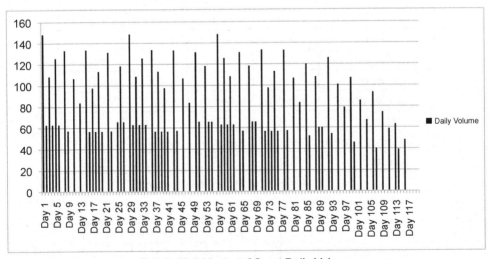

Graph 13.2 Master of Sport Daily Volume

Table 13.6 Master of Sport Daily Volume

Week	Day	Week Vol	Daily %	Day Vol
Week 1	Day 1	570	26%	148
	Day 2		11%	63
	Day 3		19%	108
	Day 4		11%	63
	Day 5		22%	125
	Day 6		11%	63
	Day 7		0%	0
Week 2	Day 8	380	35%	133
	Day 9		15%	57
	Day 10		0%	0
	Day 11		28%	106
	Day 12		0%	0
	Day 13		22%	84
	Day 14		0%	0
Week 3	Day 15	513	26%	133
	Day 16		11%	56
	Day 17		19%	97
	Day 18		11%	56
	Day 19		22%	113
	Day 20		11%	56
	Day 21		0%	0
Week 4	Day 22	437	30%	131
	Day 23		13%	57
	Day 24		0%	0
	Day 25		15%	66
	Day 26		27%	118
	Day 27		15%	66
	Day 28		0%	0
Week 5	Day 29	570	26%	148
	Day 30		11%	63
	Day 31		19%	108
	Day 32		11%	63
	Day 33		22%	125
	Day 34		11%	63
	Day 35		0%	0

Week 6	Day 36	513	26%	133
	Day 37		11%	56
	Day 38		22%	113
	Day 39		11%	56
	Day 40		19%	97
	Day 41		11%	56
	Day 42		0%	0
Week 7	Day 43	380	35%	133
	Day 44		15%	57
	Day 45		0%	0
	Day 46		28%	106
	Day 47		0%	0
	Day 48		22%	84
	Day 49		0%	0
Week 8	Day 50	437	30%	131
	Day 51		15%	66
	Day 52		0%	0
	Day 53		27%	118
	Day 54		15%	66
	Day 55		15%	66
	Day 56		0%	0
Week 9	Day 57	570	26%	148
	Day 58		11%	63
	Day 59		22%	125
	Day 60		11%	63
	Day 61		19%	108
	Day 62		11%	63
	Day 63		0%	0
Week 10	Day 64	437	30%	131
	Day 65		13%	57
	Day 66		0%	0
	Day 67		27%	118
	Day 68		15%	66
	Day 69		15%	66
	Day 70		0%	0

Week 11	Day 71	513	26%	133
	Day 72		11%	56
	Day 73		19%	97
	Day 74		11%	56
	Day 75		22%	113
	Day 76		11%	56
	Day 77		0%	0
Week 12	Day 78	380	35%	133
	Day 79		15%	57
	Day 80		0%	0
	Day 81		28%	106
	Day 82		0%	0
	Day 83		22%	84
	Day 84		0%	0
Week 13	Day 85	399	30%	120
	Day 86		13%	52
	Day 87		0%	0
	Day 88		27%	108
	Day 89		15%	60
	Day 90		15%	60
	Day 91		0%	0
Week 14	Day 92	359	35%	126
	Day 93		15%	54
	Day 94		0%	0
	Day 95		28%	101
	Day 96		0%	0
	Day 97		22%	79
	Day 98		0%	0
Week 15	Day 99	305	35%	107
	Day 100		15%	46
	Day 101		0%	0
	Day 102		28%	85
	Day 103		0%	0
	Day 104		22%	67
	Day 105		0%	0

Week 16	Day 106	266	35%	93
	Day 107		15%	40
	Day 108		0%	0
	Day 109		28%	74
	Day 110		0%	0
	Day 111		22%	59
	Day 112		0%	0
Week 17	Day 113	150	42%	63
	Day 114		26%	39
	Day 115		0%	0
	Day 116		32%	48
	Day 117		0%	0
	Day 118		0%	0
	Day 119		0%	0

SAMPLE MASTER OF SPORT TRAINING PROGRAM

The numbers to the right represent respectively the exercise volume, the daily volume and the running weekly volume. On days in which the daily volume exceeds 100 repetitions, the training has been divided up into 2 sessions in order to allow for better performance of the lifts in the second session. The first session should take place in the morning after the athlete has eaten breakfast. The second session should take place in the afternoon after lunch and possibly after a brief nap. The late afternoon is probably the best time for this training.

Week 1 (Preparation Mesocycle) 570 repetitions

Day 1—Monday (148 repetitions)
AM
1) Back Squat: 60%/3, 70%/3, (80%/3)5   21:21:21
2) Snatch Extension: (90%/3)5   15:36:36
3) Clean Deadlift: (85%/4)4   16:52:52

PM
4) Snatch: 60%/4, 70%/4, (75%/4)4   24:76:76
5) Clean & Jerk: 60%/4+1, 70%/4+1, (75%/4+1)4   30:106:106
6) Behind the Neck Power Jerk: (70%/3)2, (75%/3)2   12:118:118
7) Good Morning: (X/6)5   30:148:148

Day 2—Tuesday (63 Repetitions)
AM
1) Power Snatch: 60%/4, 65%/4, (70%/3)2   14:14:162
2) Power Clean & Power Jerk: 60%/4+1, 65%/4+1, (70%/3+1)2 18:32:180
3) Back Squat: 60%/3, 70%/3, (80%/3)2   12:44:192
4) Clean Extension: (85%/4)5   20:64:212

Day 3—Wednesday (108 repetitions)
AM
1) Front Squat: 60%/4, 70%/4, (80%/3)4   20:20:232
2) Clean High Pulls: (80%/4)5   20:40:252
3) Press: (X/4)4   16:56:268

PM
4) Snatch: 60%/3, 70%/3, (80%/3)4   18:74:286
5) Clean & Jerk: 60%/3+1, 70%/3+1, (80%/3+1)3   20:94:306
6) Snatch Deadlift: (100%/3)5   15:109:321

Day 4—Thursday (63 repetitions)
AM
1) Power Snatch & Overhead Squat: 60%/3+3, 65%/3+3, (70%/3+3)2   24:24:345
2) Power Clean & Power Jerk: 60%/3+3, 65%/3+3, (70%/3+3)2   24:48:369
3) Back Squat: 60%/3, 70%/3, (80%/3)3   15:63:384

Day 5—Friday (125 repetitions)
AM
1) Back Squat: 60%/4, 70%/4, (80%/3)4   18:18:402
2) Snatch High Pulls: (95%/4)5   20:38:422
3) Romanian Deadlift: (100%/4)4   16:52:438

PM
4) Snatch: 60%/3, 70%/3, (80%/2)4   14:66:452
5) Clean: 60%/3, 70%/3, (80%/2)4   14:80:466
6) Jerk off Rack: 70%/3, (80%/3)4   15:95:481
7) Good Morning: (X/6)5   30:125:511

Day 6—Saturday (63 repetitions)
PM
1) Back Squat: 60%/2, 70%/2, (80%/2)3   10:10:521
2) Snatch Deadlift: (105%/3)5   15:25:536
3) Clean Extension: (85%/3)4   12:37:548
4) Behind the Neck Push Press: 60%/4, 65%/4, (70%/3)3   17:54:565
5) Press: (X/3)4   12:66:577

Week 2 (Preparation Mesocycle) 380 repetitions

Day 8—Monday (133 repetitions)
AM
1) Back Squat: 60%/4, 70%/4, (80%/4)4   24:24:24
2) Snatch High Pull: (90%/4)5   20:44:44
3) Push Press: 60%/3, 65%/3, (70%/3)3   15:61:61

PM
4) Snatch: 60%/4, 70%/4, (80%/4)3   20:81:81
5) Clean: 60%/4, 70%/4, (80%/4)3   20:101:101
6) Jerk off Rack: 60%/3, 70%/3, (80%/3)3   15:116:116
7) Good Morning: (X/5)4   20:136:136

Day 9—Tuesday (57 repetitions)
AM
1) Back Squat: 60%/2, 70%/2, (80%/2)3   10:10:146
2) Power Snatch: 60%/4, 65%/4, (70%/4)2   16:26:162
3) Power Clean & Power Jerk: 60%/4+2, 65%/4+2, (70%/4+2)2   24:50:186
4) Press: (X/3)4   12:62:198

Day 10—Wednesday
Rest

Day 11—Thursday (106 repetitions)
AM
1) Front Squat: 60%/4, 70%/4, (80%/4)3   20:20:208
2) Clean Extension: (90%/4)4   16:36:224
3) Power Jerk: 60%/3, 65%/3, (70%/3)3   15:51:239

PM
4) Snatch: 60%/3, 70%/3, (80%/3, 85%/2)2   16:67:255
5) Clean & Jerk: 60%/3+1, 70%/3+1, (80%/3+1, 85%/2+1)2   22:89:277
6) Snatch Deadlifts (up in 10 seconds): (80%/3)5   15:104:292

Day 12—Friday
Rest

Day 13—Saturday (84 repetitions)
AM
1) Back Squat: 60%/3, 70%/3, (80%/3)2   12:12:304
2) Snatch: 60%/3, 70%/3, (80%/3)2   12:24:316
3) Clean & Jerk: 60%/3+1, 70%/3+1, (80%/3+1)2   16:40:332
4) Halting Clean Deadlift with 2 halts (80%/3)5   15:55:347
5) Behind the Neck Push Press: 60%/4, 65%/4, (70%/4)4   24:79:371
6) Press: (X/3)4   12:91:383

Week 3 (Preparation Mesocycle) 513 repetitions

Day 15—Monday (133 repetitions)
AM
1) Back Squat: 60%/4, 70%/4, (80%/4)5   28:28:28
2) Snatch High Pull: (95%/3)5   15:43:43
3) Press: (X/4)4   16:59:59

PM
4) Snatch: 60%/4, 70%/4, (80%/4)4   24:83:83
5) Clean: 60%/4, 70%/4, (80%/4)4   24:107:107
6) Romanian Deadlift: (100%/4)5   20:127:127

Day 16—Tuesday (56 repetitions)
AM
1) Back Squat: 60%/2, 70%/2, 80%/2, (85%/2)2   10:10:137
2) Hang Power Snatch: 60%/4, 65%/4, (70%/4)3   20:30:157
3) Hang Power Clean: 60%/4, 65%/4, (70%/4)3   20:50:177
4) Press: (X/2)4   08:58:185

Day 17—Wednesday (97 repetitions)
AM
1) Front Squat: 60%/4, 70%/4, (80%/4)5   28:28:213
2) Snatch: 60%/2, 70%/2, 80%/2, (85%/2)2   10:38:223
3) Clean & Jerk: 60%/2+2, 70%/2+2, 80%/2+2, (85%/2+2)2   20:58:243
4) Snatch Deadlifts up in 15 seconds: (80%/3)5   15:73:258
5) Good Morning: (X/6)4   24:97:282

Day 18—Thursday (56 repetitions)
AM
1) Back Squat: 60%/2, 70%/2, 80%/2, 85%/2, 90%/1   11:11:293
2) Power Snatch & Overhead Squat: 60%/3+3, (70%/3+3)3   24:35:317
3) Power Clean & Power Jerk: 60%/3+3, (70%/3+3)3   24:59:341

Day 19—Friday (113 repetitions)
AM
1) Back Squat: 60%/3, 70%/3, (80%/3)4   18:18:359
2) Snatch Extension: (95%/4)4   16:34:375
3) Clean Deadlift: (90%/3)4   12:46:387
4) Behind the Neck Push Press: 60%/4, 65%/4, (70%/4)4   24:70:411

PM
5) Hang Snatch: 60%/2, 70%/2, (80%/2)4   12:82:423
6) Hang Clean: 60%/2, 70%/2, (80%/2)4   12:94:435
7) Good Morning: (X/5)42   0:114:455

Day 20—Saturday (56 repetitions)
PM
1) Back Squat: 60%/4, 70%/4, (80%/4)2   16:16:471
2) Power Snatch: 60%/4, (70%/4)3   16:32:487
3) Power Clean & Power Jerk: 60%/4+1, (70%/4+1)3   20:52:507

Week 4 (Preparation mesocycle) 437 repetitions

Day 22—Monday (131 repetitions)
AM
1) Back Squat: 60%/2, 70%/2, (80%/4)5   24:24:24
2) Clean Extension: (85%/4)5   20:44:44
3) Power Jerk: 60%/3, 65%/3, (70%/4)3   18:62:62

PM
4) Snatch: 60%/2, 70%/2, (80%/4)4   20:82:82
5) Clean: 60%/2, 70%/2, (80%/4)3   16:98:98
6) Snatch High Pull: (100%/3)5   15:113:113
7) Clean Deadlift: (90%/4)5   20:133:133

Day 23—Tuesday (57 repetitions)
AM
1) Back Squat: 60%/2, 70%/2, 80%/2, (85%/2)3   12:12:145
2) Power Snatch: 60%/4, (70%/4)4   20:32:165
3) Power Clean: 60%/4, (70%/4)4   20:52:185
4) Press: (X/2)4   08:60:193

Day 24—Wednesday
Rest

Day 25—Thursday (66 repetitions)
AM
1) Front Squat: 60%/4, 70%/4, (80%/4)5   28:28:221
2) Push Press: 60%/4, 65%/4, (70%/4)3   20:48:241
3) Clean Deadlift (up in 10 seconds): (80%/3)6   18:66:259

Day 26—Friday (118 repetitions)
AM
1) Back Squat: 60%/3, 70%/3, 80%/3, (85%/3)4   21:21:280
2) Snatch Extension: (95%/4)5   20:41:300
3) Press: (X/3)4   12:53:312

PM
4) Hang Snatch: 60%/3, 70%/3, (80%/3)4   18:71:330
5) Hang Clean: 60%/3, 70%/3, (80%/3)3   15:86:345
6) Overhead Squat: 70%/3, (80%/3)3   12:98:357
7) Good Morning: (X/5)4   20:118:377

Day 27—Saturday (66 repetitions)
PM
1) Back Squat: 60%/2, 70%/2, 80%/2, 85%/2 90%/1   09:09:386
2) Power Snatch & Behind the Neck Push Press: 60%/3+3, (70%/3+3)3 24:35:410
3) Power Clean & Power Jerk: 60%/3+3, (70%/3+3)3   24:59:434

Week 5 (Preparation Mesocycle) 570 repetitions)

Day 29—Monday (148 repetitions)
AM
1) Back Squat: 60%/2, 70%/2, 80%/4, 85%/4, (85%/3)3   21:21:21
2) Clean High Pull: (90%/3)5   15:36:36
3) Snatch Deadlift on blocks: (100%/4)4   16:52:52
4) Behind the Neck Push Press: 60%/4, 65%/4, (70%/4)3 20:72:72

PM
5) Snatch High Pull & Snatch: 60%/3+1, 70%/3+1, (80%/3+1)4 24:96:96
6) Clean High Pull & Clean: 60%/3+1, 70%/3+1, (80%/3+1)4 24:120:120
7) Good Morning: (X/7)4   28:148:148

Day 30—Tuesday (63 repetitions)
AM
1) Back Squat: 60%/2, 70%/2, 80%/2, (85%/2)2   10:10:158
2) Power Snatch & Overhead Squat: 60%/4+4, (70%/4+4)3   32:42:190
3) Power Clean & Power Jerk: 60%/4+4, (70%/4+4)2   24:66:214

Day 31—Wednesday (108 repetitions)
AM
1) Front Squat: 60%/4, 70%/4, (80%/4)5   28:28:242
2) Snatch Extension: (100%/3)6   18:46:260

PM
3) Snatch: 60%/4, 70%/4, (80%/4)6   32:78:292
4) Clean & Jerk: 60%/4+1, 70%/4+1, (80%/4+1)5   35:113:327

Day 32—Thursday (63 repetitions)
AM
1) Back Squat: 60%/2, 70%/2, (80%/2)4   12:12:339
2) Power Snatch & Behind the Neck Push Press & Overhead Squat:
       60%/3+3+3, 65%/3+3+3, (70%/3+3+3)3   45:57:384

Day 33—Friday (125 repetitions)
AM
1) Back Squat: 60%/4, 70%/4, (80%/4, 85%/2)3   26:26:410
2) Clean Extension: (90%/4)6   24:50:434
3) Snatch Deadlift on Block: (95%/4)4   16:66:450

PM
4) Snatch: 60%/3, 70%/3, (80%/3)2, (85%/3)2   18:84:468
5) Clean & Jerk: 60%/3+1, 70%/3+1, (80%/3+1)2, (85%/3+1)2 24:108:492
6) Press: (X/4)4   16:124:508

Day 34—Saturday (63 repetitions)
PM
1) Back Squat: 60%/2, 70%/2, (80%/2)5   14:14:522
2) Power Clean & Front Squat & Jerk: 60%/3+3+3,
       65%/3+3+3, (70%/3+3+3)3   45:59:567

Week 6 (Preparation Mesocycle) 513 repetitions

Day 36—Monday (133 repetitions)
AM
1) Back Squat: 60%/4, 70%/4, 80%/4, (85%/4)3   24:24:24
2) Clean Extension: (95%/3)5   15:39:39
3) Snatch Deadlift: (100%+10 Kg/4)5   20:59:59

PM
4) Snatch: 60%/4, 70%/4, (80%/4, 85%/1)4   28:87:87
5) Clean: 60%/4, 70%/4, (80%/4, 85%/1)4   28:115:115
6) Jerk off Rack: 70%/3, 80%/3, (85%/3)4   18:133:133

Day 37—Tuesday (56 repetitions)
AM
1) Back Squat: 60%/2, 70%/2, 80%/2, (85%/2)3   12:12:145
2) Power Snatch: 60%/4, (70%/4)2, (75%/2)2   16:28:161
3) Power Clean & Power Jerk: 60%/4+2, (70%/4+2)2, (75%/2+2)2   26:54:187

Day 38—Wednesday (113 repetitions)
AM
1) Front Squat: 60%/4, 70%4, (80%/4)2, (85%/3)3   25:25:212
2) Snatch High Pull: (100%/3)5   15:40:227
3) Clean Extension: (95%/3)5   15:55:242

PM
4) Snatch: 60%/2, 70%/2, 80%/2, (85%/2)4   14:69:256
5) Clean & Jerk: 60%/2+2, 70%/2+2, 80%/2+2, (85%/2+2)4   28:97:284
6) Press: (X/4)4   16:113:300

Day 39—Thursday (56 repetitions)
AM
1) Back Squat: 60%/2, 70%/2, 80%/2, (85%/2)4   14:14:314
2) Power Snatch & Overhead Squat: 60%/3+3, 65%/3+3, (70%/3+3)5   42:56:356

Day 40—Friday (97 repetitions)
AM
1) Back Squat: 60%/4, 70%/4, (80%/4)6   32:32:388
2) Roumanian Deadlift: (95%/5)5   25:57:413

PM
3) Snatch: 60%/2, 70%/2, (80%/2)3   10:67:423
4) Clean & Jerk: 60%/2+2, 70%/2+2, (80%/2+1)3   17:84:440
5) Press: (X/3)4   12:96:452

Day 41—Saturday (56 repetitions)
PM
1) Back Squat: 60%/3, 70%/3, 80%/3, 85%/3   12:12:464
2) Power Snatch: 60%/3, 65%/3, (70%/3)2, (75%/2)3   18:30:482
3) Power Clean: 60%/3, 65%/3, (70%/3)2, (75%/2)3   18:48:490
4) Good Morning: (X/5)4   20:68:510

Week 7 (Preparation Mesocycle) 380 repetitions

Day 43 (133 repetitions)
AM
1) Back Squat: 60%/2, 70%/2, 80%/2, (85%/4)5   26:26:26
2) Snatch High Pull: (95%/3)6   18:44:44

PM
3) Snatch High Pull & Snatch: 60%/3+1, 70%/3+1,
     80%/3+1, (85%/3+1)5   32:76:76
4) Clean High Pull & Clean: 60%/3+1, 70%/3+1, 80%/3+1, (85%/3+1)4   28:104:104
5) Push Press: 60%/4, 65%/4, (70%/4)3   20:124:124

Day 44 (57 repetitions)
A M
1) Back Squat: 60%/2, 70%/2, (80%/2)2   08:08:132
2) Power Snatch: 60%/2, 65%/2, 70%/2, (75%/2)3   12:20:144
3) Power Clean: 60%/2, 65%/2, 70%/2, (75%/2)3   12:32:156
4) Clean Extension: (95%/4)5   20:52:176
5) Press: (X/3)6   18:70:194

Day 45
Rest

Day 46 (106 repetitions)
AM
1) Front Squat: 60%/2, 70%/2, 80%/2, (85%/4)5   26:26:220
2) Clean High Pull: (90%/4)5   20:46:240

PM
3) Snatch: 60%/3, 70%/3, (80%/3, 90%/1)4   22:68:262
4) Clean & Jerk: 60%/3+1, 70%/3+1, (80%/3+1, 90%/1+1)4   32:100:294
5) Press: (X/2)4   08:108:312

Day 47
Rest

Day 48 (84 repetitions)
PM
1) Back Squat: 60%/3, 70%/3, (80%/3)5   21:21:333
2) Power Snatch & Behind the Neck Push Press & Overhead Squat:
     60%/3+3+3, (70%/3+3+3)3   36:57:369
3) Power Clean & Front Squat & Power Jerk:
     60%/3+3+3, (70%/3+3+3)3   36:87:405

Week 8 (Preparation mesocycle) 437 repetitions

Day 50—Monday (131 repetitions)
AM
1) Back Squat: 60%/2, 70%/2, 80%/2, (85%/4)6   30:30:30
2) Snatch Extension: (100%/4)5   20:50:50

PM
3) Snatch: 60%/2, 70%/2, 80%/2, (85%/4)3   18:68:68
4) Clean: 60%/2, 70%/2, 80%/2, (85%/4)3   18:86:86
5) Jerk off rack: 60%/2, 70%/2, 80%/2, (85%/3)3   15:101:101
6) Clean High Pull: (95%/3)5   15:116:116
7) Press: (X/3)5   15:131:131

Day 51—Tuesday (66 repetitions)
AM
1) Power Snatch & Overhead Squat: 60%/4+4, 65%/4+4, (70%/4+4)3   40:40:171
2) Power Clean & Power Jerk: 60%/3+3, 65%/3+3, (70%/3+3)2   24:64:195

Day 52—Wednesday
Rest

Day 53—Thursday (118 repetitions)
AM
1) Front Squat: 60%/2, 70%/2, 80%/2, (85%/4)5   26:26:221
2) Clean Extension: (90%/5)5   25:51:246

PM
3) Snatch: 60%/3, 70%/3, (80%/3)4   18:69:264
4) Clean & Jerk: 60%/1+3, 70%/1+3, (80%/1+3)4   24:93:288
5) Snatch High Pull: (95%/4)6   24:117:312

Day 54—Friday (66 repetitions)
AM
1) Back Squat: 60%/3, 70%/3, (80%/3)5   21:21:333
2) Power Snatch: 60%/3, 65%/3, (70%/3)4   18:39:351
3) Power Clean & Power Jerk: 60%/4+4, 65%/4+4, (70%/4+4)2   32:71:383

Day 55—Saturday (66 repetitions)
PM
1) Back Squat: 60%/2, 70%/2, (80%/4)2, (85%/4)2   24:24:409
2) Snatch Extension: (95%/4)4   16:40:423
3) Good Morning: (X/6)4   24:64:447

Week 9 (Preparation Mesocycle) 570 repetitions

Day 57—Monday (148 repetitions)
AM
1) Back Squat: 60%/2, 70%/2, 80%/2, (85%/4)6	30:30:30
2) Snatch High Pull: (90%/5)5	25:55:55
3) Clean Deadlift: (100%/3)4	12:62:62
4) Press: (X/4)5	20:82:82

PM
5) Snatch: 60%/2, 70%/2, 80%/2, (85%/4)5	26:108:108
6) Clean: 60%/2, 70%/2, 80%/2, (85%/4)4	22:130:130
7) Good Morning: (X/5)4	20:150:150

Day 58—Tuesday (63 repetitions)
AM
1) Back Squat: 60%/2, 70%/2, 80%/2, (85%/2)5	16:16:166
2) Power Snatch: 60%/3, 70%/3, 75%/2, 70%/2, 75%/1	11:27:177
3) Power Clean & Power Jerk: 60%/3+2, 70%/3+1, 75%/2+1, 70%/2+1, 75%/1+1	17:44:194
4) Push Press: 60%/4, 65%/4, (70%/4)3	20:64:214

Day 59—Wednesday (125 repetitions)
AM
1) Front Squat: 60%/2, 70%/2, 80%/2, (85%/4)6	30:30:244
2) Clean Extension: (95%/3)5	15:45:259
3) Press: (X/4)5	20:65:279

PM
4) Snatch: 60%/3, 70%/3, (80%/3)6	24:89:303
5) Clean & Jerk: 60%/1+3, 70%/1+3, (80%/1+3)3, (85%/1+3)2	28:117:331
6) Snatch Extension: (105%/2)4	08:125:339

Day 60—Thursday (63 repetitions)
AM
1) Power Snatch: 60%/4, 65%/4, (70%/4, 75%/1)3	23:23:362
2) Power Clean & Power Jerk: 60%/4+2, 65%/4+2, (70%/4+2, 75%/1+2)3	39:62:401

Day 61—Friday (108 repetitions)
AM
1) Back Squat: 60%/3, 70%/3, 80%/3, 85%/3, 90%/1	13:13:414
2) Snatch High Pull: (105%/3)5 15:28:429	
3) Power Jerk: 60%/4, 65%/4, 70%/4, 75%/3, (70%/4)2	23:51:452

PM
4) Snatch High Pull & Snatch: 60%/3+1, 70%/3+1, (80%/3+1)5	28:79:480
5) Clean High Pull & Clean: 60%/3+1, 70%/3+1, (80%/3+1)4	24:103:504
6) Press: (X/3)4	12:115:516

Day 62—Saturday (63 repetitions)
AM
1) Back Squat: 60%/2, 70%/2, 80%/2, (85%/4)5   26:26:542
2) Clean Extension: (95%/4)5   20:46:562

PM
3) Snatch: 60%/2, 70%/2, 80%/2, (85%/2)4   14:60:576
4) Clean: 60%/2, 70%/2, 80%/2, (85%/2)3   12:72:588

Week 10 (Preparation mesocycle) 437 repetitions

Day 64—Monday (131 repetitions)
AM
1) Back Squat: 60%/2, 70%/2, 80%/2, (85%/4, 90%/1)4   26:26:26
2) Clean High Pull: (95%/4)6   24:50:50
3) Push Press: 60%/3, 70%/3, (75%/2)2, 70%/3   13:63:63

PM
4) Snatch: 60%/3, 70%/3, (80%/3)2, (85%/3)4   24:87:87
5) Clean & Jerk: 60%/1+3, 70%/1+3, (80%/1+3)2, (85%/1+3)4   32:119:119
6) Press: (X/3)4   12:131:131

Day 65—Tuesday (57 repetitions)
AM
1) Back Squat: 60%/2, 70%/2, (80%/2/)2, (85%/2)2   12:12:143
2) Snatch Extension: (105%/3)6   18:30:161
3) Romanian Deadlift: (95%/5)5   25:55:186

Day 66—Wednesday
Rest

Day 67—Thursday (118 repetitions)
AM
1) Front Squat: 60%/2 70%/2, 80%/2, (85%/4, 90%/1)4   26:26:212
2) Clean Extension: 90%/4, (95%/4)5   24:50:236
3) Power Jerk: 60%/2, 65%/4, (70%/4, 75%/2)3   24:74:260

PM
4) Power Snatch: 60%/,2 65%/2, (70%/4, 75%/2)3   22:96:282
5) Power Clean: 60%/2, 65%/2, (70%/4, 75%/2)3   22:118:304

Day 68—Friday (66 repetitions)
AM
1) Back Squat: 60%/2, 70%/2, (80%/2), (85%/2)2   12:12:316
2) Snatch Extension: (105%/3)6   18:30:334
3) Press: (X/4)4   16:46:350
4) Good Morning: (X/5)4   20:66:370

Day 69—Saturday (66 repetitions)
PM
1) Front Squat: 60%/3, 70%/3, 80%/3, 85%/3   12:12:382
2) Snatch: 60%/3, 70%/3, 80%/3, 85%/3   12:24:394
3) Clean & Jerk: 60%/3+1, 70%/3+1, 80%/3+1, 85%/3+1   16:40:410
4) Clean Extension: (95%/3)5   15:55:425
5) Push Press: 60%/3, 65%/3, 70%/3, 75%/2   11:66:426

Week 11 (Preparation Mesocycle) 513 repetitions

Day 71—Monday (133 repetitions)
AM
1) Back Squat: 60%/2, 70%/2, (80%/4, 85%/4, 90%/1)3   31:31:31
2) Clean High Pull: (95%/4)5   20:51:51
3) Push Press: 60%/2, 65%/2, (70%/4, 75%/2)3   22:73:73

PM
4) Snatch: 60%/2, 70%/2, (80%/4, 85%/3)3   25:98:98
5) Clean: 60%/2, 70%/2, (80%/4, 85%/3)3   25:123:123
6) Press: (X/3)4   12:135:135

Day 72—Tuesday (56 repetitions)
AM
1) Back Squat: 60%/2, 70%/2, 80%/2, (85%/2)4   14:14:149
2) Power Snatch & Overhead Squat: 60%/3+4, 65%/3+4, (70%/3+4)3   35:49:184
3) Power Clean: 60%/2, 65%/2, (70%/2)2   08:57:192

Day 73—Wednesday (97 repetitions)
PM
1) Front Squat: 60%/2, 70%/2, (80%/4, 85%/4, 90%/1)3   31:31:223
2) Snatch: 60%/2, 70%/2, 80%/2, (85%/4)4   22:53:245
3) Clean: 60%/2, 70%/2, 80%/2, (85%/2)4   22:75:267
4) Jerk off Rack: 60%/2, 70%/2, 80%/2, (85%/3)5   21:96:289

Day 74—Thursday (56 repetitions)
AM
1) Back Squat: 60%/2, 70%/2, 80%/2, 85%/2, 90%/1, 95%/1   10:10:299
2) Power Snatch: 60%/3, 65%/3, 70%/3, (75%/3)3   18:28:317
3) Power Clean & Power Jerk: 60%/3+2, 70%/3+2, (75%/3+2)3   25:53:342

Day 75—Friday (113 repetitions)
AM
1) Back Squat: 60%/2, 70%/2, 80%/2, 85%/2, (90%/2)5   18:18:360
2) Snatch: 60%/2, 70%/2, 80%/2, 85%/2, 80%/4, 85%/3   15:33:375
3) Clean & Jerk: 60%/2+1, 70%/2+1, 80%/2+1, 85%/2+1,
      80%/4+1, 85%/3+1   21:54:396

PM
4) Snatch Extension: (105%/3)6   18:72:414
5) Clean Deadlift: (105%/3)5   15:92:429
6) Good Morning: (X/6)4   24:116:453

Day 76—Saturday (56 repetitions)
PM
1) Front Squat: 60%/2, 70%/2, 80%/2, (85%/2)4   14:14:467
2) Power Snatch: 60%/2, 70%/2, (75%/2, 80%/1)3   13:27:480
3) Power Clean & Power Jerk: 60%/2+2, 70%/2+2,
        (75%/2+2, 80%/1+1)3   26:53:506

Week 12 (Preparation Mesocycle) 380 Repetitions

Day 78: Monday (133 repetitions)
AM
1) Back Squat: 60%/2, 70%/2, 80%/2, (85%/4)4   22:22:22
2) Snatch Extension: (105%/3)5   15:37:37
3) Press: (X/4)4   16:53:53

PM
4) Snatch: 60%/2, 70%/2, 80%/2, (85%/3, 90%/1)5   26:79:79
5) Clean: 60%/2, 70%/2, 80%/2, (85%/3, 90%/1)4   22:101:101
6) Clean High Pull: (100%/3)4   12:113:113
7) Power Jerk: 60%/2, 70%/2, (75%/4)4   20:133:133

Day 79—Tuesday (57 repetitions)
AM
1) Back Squat: 60%/2, 70%/2, 80%/2, 85%/2, 90%/2   10:10:143
2) Power Snatch: 60%/2, 70%/2, (75%/3)3   13:23:156
3) Power Clean & Power Jerk: 60%/2+2, 70%/2+2, (75%/3+2)3 23:46:179
4) Snatch High Pull: (105%/3)4   12:58:191

Day 80—Wednesday
Rest

Day 81—Thursday (106 repetitions)
AM
1) Front Squat: 60%/2, 70%/2, 80%/2, (85%/4)4   22:22:213
2) Clean Extension: (100%/3)5   15:37:228
3) Push Press: 60%/4, 70%/4, (75%/3)4   20:57:248

PM
4) Snatch: 60%/2, 70%/2, 80%/2, 85%/2, 90%/1, 95%/1, (85%/2)3   16:73:264
5) Clean & Jerk: 60%/2+1, 70%/2+1, 80%/2+1, 85%/2+1,
        90%/1+1, 95%/1+1, (85%/2+1)3   25:98:289
6) Press: (X/2)4   08:106:297

Day 82—Friday
Rest

Day 83—Saturday (84 repetitions)
PM
1) Back Squat: 60%/2, 70%/2, 80%/2, 85%/3, 90%/2, 95%/1, (85%/3)3   21:21:318
2) Snatch: 60%/2, 70%/2, 80%/2, 85%/3, 90%/2, 95%/1, (85%/3)3   21:42:339
3) Clean & Jerk: 60%/2+1, 70%/2+1, 80%/2+1, 85%/3+1,
       90%/1+1, 95%/1+1, (85%/3+1)3   30:72:369
4) Good Morning: (X/5)4   20:92:389

Week 13 (Pre-Competition Mesocycle) 399 repetitions

Day 85—Monday (120 Repetitions)
AM
1) Snatch: 60%/2, 70%/2, 80%/2, 85%/2, (90%/2)5   18:18:18
2) Clean & Jerk: 60%/2+1, 70%/2+1, 80%/2+1, 85%/2+1, (90%/2+1)4   24:42:42
3) Snatch Extension: (105%/2)6   12:54:54

PM
4) Back Squat: 60%/1, 70%/1, 80%/1, (85%/3, 90%/2, 95%/1)3   21:75:75
5) Power Jerk: 60%/2, 70%/2, (75%/2, 80%/1)3   13:88:88
6) Press: (X/4)4   16:104:104
7) Good Morning: (X/5)4   20:124:124

Day 86—Tuesday (52 repetitions)
AM
1) Power Snatch: 60%/2, 70%/2, (75%/2, 80%/1)3   13:13:137
2) Power Clean & Power Jerk: 60%/2+1, 70%/2+1,
       (75%/2+1, 80%/1+1)3   21:34:158
3) Clean Deadlift: (105%/3)6   18:52:176

Day 87—Wednesday
Rest

Day 88—Thursday (108 repetitions)
AM
1) Snatch: 60%/1, 70%/1, 80%/1, 85%/1, 90%/1, (95%/1)4   09:09:185
2) Clean & Jerk: 60%/1+1, 70%/1+1, 80%/1+1, 85%/1+1,
       90%/1+1, (95%/1+1)4   18:27:203
3) Snatch Deadlift: (110%/2)6   12:39:215
4) Front Squat: 60%/1, 70%/1, 80%/1, 85%/1, 90%/1, (95%/1)5   10:49:225

PM
5) Clean Extension: (100%/3)6   18:67:243
6) Push Press: 60%/3, 65%/3, (70%/3, 75%/2, 80%/1)3   24:91:267
7) Good Morning: (X/4)4   16:107:283

Day 89—Friday (60 repetitions)
AM
1) Power Snatch: 60%/2, 70%/2, (75%/2, 80%/1)3   13:13:296
2) Power Clean & Power Jerk: 60%/2+2, 70%/2+2,
      (75%/2+2, 80%/1+1)3   26:39:322
3) Snatch Extension: (105%/3)4   12:51:334
4) Press: (X/2)4   08:59:342

Day 90—Saturday (60 repetitions)
PM
1) Snatch: 60%/2, 70%/2, 80%/2, 85%/2, (90%/2)3   14:14:358
2) Clean & Jerk: 60%/2+1, 70%/2+1, 80%/2+1, 85%/2+1, (90%/2+1)3   21:35:379
3) Front Squat: 60%/2, 70%/2, 80%/2, 85%/2, (90%/2)3   14:49:393

Week 14 (Pre-Competition Mesocycle): 359 repetitions

Day 92—Monday (126 repetitions)
AM
1) Front Squat: 60%/2, 70%/2, 80%/2, 85%/2 (90%/2)5   18:18:18
2) Snatch Extensions: (105%/2)6   12:30:30
3) Power Jerk: 60%/2, 70%/2, (75%/3, 80%/2)3   19:49:49

PM
4) Snatch: singles to max, (max-10, max-5, max)3   17:66:66
5) Clean & Jerk: singles to max, (max-10, max-5, max)3   34:100:100
6) Good Morning: (X/5)5   25:125:125

Day 93—Tuesday (54 repetitions)
AM
1) Power Snatch: singles to max (max-10, max-5, max)3   13:13:138
2) Power Clean & Jerk: singles to max, (max-10, max-5, max)3   26:39:164
3) Clean Extensions: (100%/3)3, (105%/3)3   18:57:182

Day 94—Wednesday
Rest

Day 95—Thursday (101 repetitions)
AM
1) Snatch: 60%/1, 70%/1, 80%/1, 85%/1, 90%/1, 95%/1, (80%/3)4   18:18:200
2) Clean & Jerk: 60%/1+1, 70%/1+1, 80%/1+1, 85%/1+1,
      90%/1+1, 95%/1+1, (80%/3+1)3   24:42:224
3) Press: (X/3)4   12:54:236

PM
4) Back Squat: 60%/1, 70%/1, 80%/1, 85%/1, 90%/1, 95%/1, (80%/3)5   21:75:257
5) Snatch Extension: (100%/3)3, (105%/2)3   15:90:272
6) Power Jerk: 60%/2, 70%/2, 75%/2, (80%/2)3   10:100:282

Day 96—Friday
Rest

Day 97—Saturday (79 repetitions)
1) Snatch: 60%/2, 70%/2, 80%/2, (85%/2)4   14:14:296
2) Clean & Jerk: 60%/2+2, 70%/2+2, 80%/2+2, (85%/2+2)3   24:38:320
3) Clean Extension: (95%/2)3, (100%/2)4   14:52:334
4) Front Squat: 60%/2, 70%/2, 80%/2, (85%/2, 90%/1, 95%/1)3 18:70:352
5) Press: (X/2)4   08:78:360

Week 15 (Pre-competition Mesocycle) 305 repetitions

Day 99—Monday (107 repetitions)
AM
1) Snatch: Singles to max, (max-10, max-5, max)3   17:17:17
2) Clean & Jerk: Singles to max, (max-10, max-5, max)3   34:51:51

PM
3) Front Squat: Singles to max, (max-10, max-5, max)3   17:68:68
4) Snatch Extension: (105% + 10 Kg/2)6   12:80:80
5) Clean Extension: (105%/2)4   08:88:88
6) Press: (X/3)5   15:103:103

Day 100—Tuesday (46 repetitions)
1) Power Snatch: singles to max (max-10, max-5, max)3   13:13:116
2) Power Clean & Jerk: singles to max, (max-10, max-5, max)3 26:39:142
3) Snatch High Pull: (105%/2)4   08:47:150

Day 101—Wednesday
Rest

Day 102—Thursday (85 repetitions)
1) Snatch: Singles to max   08:08:158
2) Clean & Jerk: Singles to max   16:24:174
3) Clean Extension: (105%/2)6   12:36:186
4) Back Squat: singles to max, (max-10, max-5, max)4   21:57:207
5) Push Press: 60%/3, 70%/3, (75%/3)3   15:72:222
6) Snatch Deadlift: (110%/2)5   10:82:232

Day 103—Friday
Rest

Day 104—Saturday (67 repetitions)
1) Snatch: 60%/2, 70%/2, 80%/2, (85%/2)2, (90%/2)2   14:14:246
2) Clean & Jerk: 60%/2+2, 70%/2+2, 80%/2+2, (85%/2+1)2, (90%/2+1)2 24:38:270
3) Snatch Extension: (105% + 10 Kg/2)5   10:48:280
4) Front Squat: 60%/2, 70%/2, 80%/2, (85%/2)2, (90%/2)2   14:62:294
5) Press: (X/2)4   08:70:302

Week 16 (Pre-competition Mesocycle) 266 repetitions

Day 106—Monday (93 repetitions)
1) Snatch: singles to max, (max-10, max-5, max)2	14:14:14
2) Clean & Jerk: singles to max, (max-10, max-5, max)2	28:42:42
3) Snatch Extension: (100%/2)5	10:52:52
4) Front Squat: singles to max, (max-10, max-5, max)2	14:66:66
5) Good Morning: (X/5)4	20:86:86
6) Press: (X/2)4	08:94:94

Day 107—Tuesday (40 repetitions)
1) Power Snatch: singles to max (max-10, max-5, max)2	10:10:104
2) Power Clean & Jerk: singles to max, (max-10, max-5, max)2	20:30:124
3) Clean Deadlift: (100%/2)5	10:40:134

Day 108—Wednesday
Rest

Day 109—Thursday (74 repetitions)
1) Snatch: singles to max, (90%/2)3	14:14:148
2) Clean & Jerk: singles to max (90%/2+1)3	25:39:173
3) Back Squat: singles to max (90%/2)3	14:53:187
4) Clean Extension: (95%/2)6	12:65:199
5) Press: (X/2)4	08:73:207

Day 110—Friday
Rest

Day 111—Saturday (59 repetitions)
1) Snatch: 60%/2, 70%/2, 80%/2, (85%/2)3	12:12:219
2) Clean & Jerk: 60%/2+1, 70%/2+1, 80%/2+1, (85%/2+1)3	18:30:237
3) Snatch Extension: (95%/3)4	12:42:249
4) Front Squat: 60%/2, 70%/2, 80%/2, (85%/2)2, (90%/2)2	14:56:263

Day 112—Sunday
Rest

Week 17 (Pre-competition Mesocycle) 150 Repetitions

Day 113—Monday (47 repetitions)
AM
1) Snatch: 60%/1, 70%/1, 80%/1, 85%/1, 90%/1, 95%/1, 85%/1, 90%/1	08:08:08
2) Clean & Jerk: 60%/1+1, 70%/1+1, 80%/1+1, 85%/1+1, 90%/1+1, 95%/1+1, 85%/1+1, 90%/1+1	16:24:24
3) Snatch Extension: (95%/2)4	08:32:32
4) Front Squat: 60%/2, 70%/2, 80%/2, 85%/2, 90%/1, 80%/2, 85%/2	13:45:45

Day 114—Tuesday (39 repetitions)
PM
1) Power Snatch: 60%/2, 65%/2, 70%/2, (75%/1)3   12:12:57
2) Power Clean & Jerk: 60%/2+2, 65%/2+2, 70%/2+2, (75%/1+1)3   18:30:75
3) Press: (X/2)4   08:38:83

Day 115—Wednesday
Rest

Day 116—Thursday (48 repetitions)
1) Power Snatch: 60%/2, (70%/2)3   08:08:91
2) Power Clean & Jerk: 60%/2+1, (70%/2+1)3   12:20:103
3) Jumping Back Squat: (50%/2)4   08:28:111
4) Push Press: 60%/2, 65%/2, (70%/2)2   08:36:119

Day 117—Friday
Rest

Day 118—Saturday
Competition

CHAPTER 14
INTERNATIONAL MASTER OF SPORT

The International Master of Sport is the highest classification. It is based on the average of 8th place at the world championships and Olympic Games of the preceding quadrennium. If one is to consider the qualifying totals for this class to be 100% figures, the percentage gap between this class and the next lowest one (Master of Sport) is the greatest. The percentage difference here is approximately 20%, whereas the differences between the lower classes are in the single digits.

This means that talent plays a great part in determining in which class an athlete is to eventually find him or herself. IMS weightlifters are considered professionals and are paid enough to be able to accommodate the many time demands of training for the IMS standards. These lifters are trained by professional coaches and in all probability in a team setting where other athletes help to form the human psychic ambience. They are also able to access restoration facilities and personnel, as well as sports medicine professionals, sports nutritionists, sports psychologists and other specialists as needed.

They have already represented their nations at world or continental junior championships, and at the very least, minor international competitions. They have mastered the art of weightlifting preparation and performance from the athlete's perspective and they are driven to complete a career as a professional athlete before age limits the restorational capacities.

The International Master of Sports qualifying totals for men are shown in Table 14.1. The International Master of Sports qualifying totals for women are shown in Table 14.2.

Weight Class (kg)	56	62	69	77	85	94	105	+105
Total (kg)	255	285	320	350	365	385	400	415

Table 14.1 International Master of Sport Men Qualification

Weight Class (kg)	48	53	58	63	69	75	+75
Totals (kg)	165	180	190	205	215	225	235

Table 14.2 International Master of Sport Women Qualification

The training volumes for athletes in this category are exceptionally high, although they are modified somewhat to accommodate older and heavier athletes. The average intensity is very high, with most of the intensities at 80% and above. This is especially demanding and cannot be accomplished without the support of proper restoration. The amount of time occupied in the daily schedule by restoration and sports medicine prohibits the athlete from doing very much other than being involved in the preparatory process. Proper nutrition plays a great part as well in terms of nourishing the organism and ensuring that nutrients are available to repair the tissues that are broken down through the training process. This includes the adequate supply of vitamins, minerals and other micronutrients that facilitate the various metabolic processes that must be accelerated in order to train in a demanding manner over prolonged periods.

This level of coaching also requires that the coach manage the various aspects of the athlete's regimen. The organization of the daily schedule to accommodate training, restoration, and feeding must occupy a significant amount of the coach's time, and as a result, each coach cannot be directly responsible for more than four lifters during a period that extends over several macrocycles.

Exercise Selection

The exercises to be employed are the same as those employed for the Master of Sport Class. The exercises are geared toward developing strength in an individual and to maintaining and increasing dynamic characteristics. There will be fewer pulling movements performed from the various hang heights and from blocks. Those that are performed will take place during the preparation mesocycles. There will be very few partial movements unless the athlete is returning from an injury. The proportion of classical lifts and their derivatives to strength building exercises will vary considerably between the preparation mesocycles and the pre-competition mesocycles.

The loading will be the primary variant rather than the exercise choices. Some of these exercises will be employed only in the event of a need for remediation, and then will be discontinued once the weakness is brought into balance. Again, the variety of exercises will diminish as the competition draws near. *On blocks* means the lifter is standing on a block that places the instep very nearly touching the bar at the starting position. *Off blocks* means that the bar is resting on blocks that elevate it off the floor at varied heights prior to the start of each repetition.

The 18 Most Appropriate Exercises To Be Included In the Training Program of an International Master of Sport Lifter:

1) Snatch (from the hang, on blocks, off blocks)
2) Clean & Jerk
3) Cleans (from the hang, on blocks, off blocks)
4) Jerk off Rack
5) Power Snatch (from the hang, on blocks, off blocks)
6) Power Clean (from the hang, on blocks, off blocks)
7) Power Jerk (in combination with power cleans or off racks)
8) Snatch Pull (or Extension, on blocks, off blocks)

9) Clean Pull (or Extension, on blocks, off blocks)

10) Snatch Deadlift (Halting, Slow and Eccentric, on blocks)

11) Clean Deadlift (Halting, Slow and Eccentric, on blocks)

12) Romanian Deadlift (May be on blocks)

13) Back Squat (Halting, Slow and Eccentric)

14) Front Squat (Halting, Slow and Eccentric)

15) Push Press (off rack)

16) Press (Standing, Seated or Supine on flat or incline bench)

17) Good Mornings (Straight-legged or bent-legged)

18) Overhead Squat

Yearly Loading Parameters

The goal of this training is to elevate the performance level of exceptional weightlifters up to international caliber. Almost all athletes that reach this class ranking have progressed through the previous ranks very rapidly due to their talent. At this point all the physical factors should be in place to embark on the most strenuous training regimen.

The annual training volume for an International Master of Sport lies within the 20,000 to 25,000 range with variation being determined by age and bodyweight factors. The number of repetitions in the 90%—100% range for snatch and clean & jerk lifts is from 400—700 for the year. Again, the cleans and the jerks are counted as separate repetitions.

The relative intensity range for snatch and clean & jerk exercises normally falls in the 73%—77% range. This figure may be skewed by the practice of including power snatches, power cleans and power jerks. Typically a well-balanced, thoroughly-trained weightlifter will have 100% figures in these lifts that are approximately 80% of the maximum for the classic versions. This means that if an athlete has a maximum classic snatch of 160 kg, and the maximum power snatch is 80% of that (128 kg), then a 64% of classic snatch weight is 102.4 kg and is counted in terms of relative intensity as 80% of the power snatch figure. The manner in which relative intensity is determined will then affect this relative intensity range.

The average volume for a four-week preparation mesocycle for International Masters has been calculated at 2,360 repetitions. The volume for a pre-competition mesocycle drops down to 1,500 repetitions. The maximum number of hours spent in training should range from 34 to 36 hours.

Loading in Zones of Intensity: Distribution of Year Volume

The percentages in Table 14.3 represent the percentage of the annual volume for the exercise group designated in the first column. Remember that these are empirically derived guideline numbers that have proven to be effective. They are most useful when they are considered representatives of trends and patterns. They can and should be modified by an experienced coach.

Intensity	50-55%	60-65%	70-75%	80-85%	90-95%	100-105%	110%	Yearly Average
Snatch Exercises		16%	63%	19%	2%			71%
Clean & Jerk Exercises		11%	55%	31%		3%		73%
Snatch Pull				25%	37%	32%	6%	91%
Clean Pull			20%	38%	24%	13%	5%	84%
Squats	22%	30%	25%	20%	2%			66%
Fundamental Exercises	4%	13%	39%	25%	10%	8%	1%	79%

Table 14.3 International Master of Sport Zones of Intensity
*Does not include good mornings or presses

The snatch exercises include all snatches and power snatches. Clean & jerk exercises include all cleans, power cleans, jerks and power jerks. The numbers for squat exercises has probably shifted toward the right. Higher intensity squats are valuable for generally strengthening the body and only in extreme cases should the average intensities be reduced if they are affecting the development of speed characteristics. Again, the calculation of the figures for squats may be skewed by including overhead squats into this group and employing the absolute weights in the calculations. The Fundamental Exercises include all exercises in Groups 1—10 as listed in Chapter 8.

Calculations

For International Master of Sport athletes, it is advisable to schedule the major peak competition after three four-week preparation mesocycles followed by a five-week pre-competition mesocycle. This means that the weekly volumes must be varied during the preparation phase so that they do fall into a regular pattern and can build up to a high volume point that sufficiently taxes the endocrines. The percentage of the 2,360 repetitions of the preparation mesocycle and the 1,500 repetitions of the pre-competition mesocycle given over to the four weeks are 30%, 27%, 23% and 20% in any order. (Table 14.4)

Prep Month 1	Week 1	Week 2	Week 3	Week 4
Volume	708	542	637	472
Prep Month 2	Week 5	Week 6	Week 7	Week 8
Volume	708	637	472	542
Prep Month 3	Week 9	Week 10	Week 11	Week 12
Volume	708	542	637	472
Pre-Comp Month	Week 13	Week 14	Week 15	Week 16
Volume	450	345	405	300

Table 14.4 International Master of Sport Weekly Volume

A 17th tapering week should precede the competition. The volume should be approximately 150 repetitions. This is therefore a 17-week cycle. The data from Table 14.4 is represented in Graph 14.1.

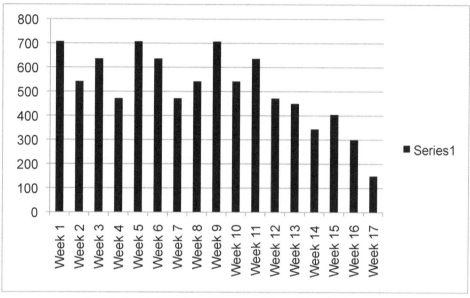

Graph 14.1 International Master of Sport Weekly Volumes

The training volume is then apportioned into the number of training days per week. (Table 14.5)

Week	1	2	3	4	5	6	7	8	9	10	11	12	13	14	15	16	17
Training Days	6	6	6	6	6	6	6	6	6	6	6	6	6	5	5	4	3

Table 14.5 International Master of Sport Training Days per Week

Table 14.6 and Graph 14.2 show the daily volumes for a 17-Week macrocycle for an International Master of Sport weightlifter. The preparation mesocycles are highlighted in gray.

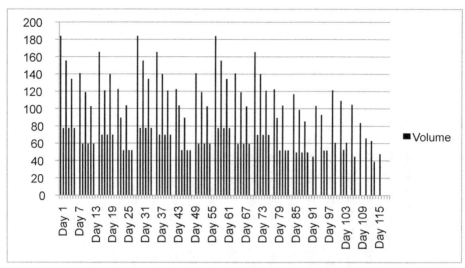

Graph 14.2 International Master of Sport Training Daily Volumes

Table 14.6 International Master of Sport Daily Volume

Week	Day	Week Vol	Daily %	Day Vol
Week 1	Day 1	708	26%	184
	Day 2		11%	78
	Day 3		22%	156
	Day 4		11%	78
	Day 5		19%	135
	Day 6		11%	78
	Day 7		0%	0
Week 2	Day 8	542	26%	141
	Day 9		11%	60
	Day 10		22%	119
	Day 11		11%	60
	Day 12		19%	103
	Day 13		11%	60
	Day 14		0%	0
Week 3	Day 15	637	26%	166
	Day 16		11%	70
	Day 17		19%	121
	Day 18		11%	70
	Day 19		22%	140
	Day 20		11%	70
	Day 21		0%	0

Week 4	Day 22	472	26%	123
	Day 23		19%	90
	Day 24		11%	52
	Day 25		22%	104
	Day 26		11%	52
	Day 27		11%	52
	Day 28		0%	0
Week 5	Day 29	708	26%	184
	Day 30		11%	78
	Day 31		22%	156
	Day 32		11%	78
	Day 33		19%	135
	Day 34		11%	78
	Day 35		0%	0
Week 6	Day 36	637	26%	166
	Day 37		11%	70
	Day 38		22%	140
	Day 39		11%	70
	Day 40		19%	121
	Day 41		11%	70
	Day 42		0%	0
Week 7	Day 43	472	26%	123
	Day 44		22%	104
	Day 45		11%	52
	Day 46		19%	90
	Day 47		11%	52
	Day 48		11%	52
	Day 49		0%	0
Week 8	Day 50	542	26%	141
	Day 51		11%	60
	Day 52		22%	119
	Day 53		11%	60
	Day 54		19%	103
	Day 55		11%	60
	Day 56		0%	0

Week 9	Day 57	708	26%	184
	Day 58		11%	78
	Day 59		22%	156
	Day 60		11%	78
	Day 61		19%	135
	Day 62		11%	78
	Day 63		0%	0
Week 10	Day 64	542	26%	141
	Day 65		11%	60
	Day 66		22%	119
	Day 67		11%	60
	Day 68		19%	103
	Day 69		11%	60
	Day 70		0%	0
Week 11	Day 71	637	26%	166
	Day 72		11%	70
	Day 73		22%	140
	Day 74		11%	70
	Day 75		19%	121
	Day 76		11%	70
	Day 77		0%	0
Week 12	Day 78	472	26%	123
	Day 79		19%	90
	Day 80		11%	52
	Day 81		22%	104
	Day 82		11%	52
	Day 83		11%	52
	Day 84		0%	0
Week 13	Day 85	450	26%	117
	Day 86		11%	50
	Day 87		22%	99
	Day 88		11%	50
	Day 89		19%	86
	Day 90		11%	50
	Day 91		0%	0

Week 14	Day 92	345	13%	45
	Day 93		30%	104
	Day 94		0%	0
	Day 95		27%	93
	Day 96		15%	52
	Day 97		15%	52
	Day 98		0%	0
Week 15	Day 99	405	30%	122
	Day 100		15%	61
	Day 101		0%	0
	Day 102		27%	109
	Day 103		13%	53
	Day 104		15%	61
	Day 105		0%	0
Week 16	Day 106	300	35%	105
	Day 107		15%	45
	Day 108		0%	0
	Day 109		28%	84
	Day 110		0%	0
	Day 111		22%	66
	Day 112		0%	0
Week 17	Day 113	150	42%	63
	Day 114		26%	39
	Day 115		0%	0
	Day 116		32%	48
	Day 117		0%	0
	Day 118		0%	0
	Day 119			0

SAMPLE INTERNATIONAL MASTER OF SPORT TRAINING PROGRAM

This is a detailed program showing the specific exercises with accompanying appropriate percentages, repetitions and sets. The numbers in the column to the right represent respectively the exercise volume, the daily volume, and the weekly volume. The total weekly volume follows the boldfaced week designation, and the daily volume follows each day. On the days where the volume exceeds 100 repetitions, the training is divided into two sessions. The first one is after breakfast has been digested, and the second one is in the afternoon after lunch and ideally a brief nap.

Week 1 (Preparation mesocycle 1) 708 repetitions

Day 1—Monday (184 repetitions)
AM
1) Back Squat: 60%/5, 70%/5, (75%/5)5   35:35:35
2) Snatch Extension: (80%/5)5   25:60:60
3) Push Press: 60%/4, 65%/4, (70%/3)3   17:77:77

PM
4) Snatch: 60%/3, 70%/3, (80%/2)6   18:95:95
5) Clean & Jerk: 60%/3+1, 70%/3+1, (80%/2+1)6   26:121:121
6) Snatch Deadlift: (85%/5)6   30:151:151
7) Back Squat: (80%/3)4   12:163:163
8) Good Morning: (X/5)4   20:183:183

Day 2—Tuesday (78 repetitions)
AM
1) Power Snatch & Behind the Neck Push Press & Overhead Squat:
      60%/3+3+3, 65%/3+3+3, (70%/2+2+2)3   36:36:219
2) Power Clean & Front Squat & Power Jerk:
      60%/3+3+3, 65%/3+3+3, (70%/2+2+2)3   36:72:255
3) Back Squat: (80%/2)4   08:80:263

Day 3—Wednesday (156 repetitions)
1) Back Squat: 60%/2, 70%/2, (75%/5)6   34:34:289
2) Clean Extension: (80%/3)6   18:52:307
3) Snatch Deadlift: (100%/4)5   20:72:327

PM
4) Snatch: 60%/2, 70%/2, (80%/2)6   16:88:343
5) Clean & Jerk: 60%/2+2, 70%/2+2, (80%/2+1)5   23:111:366
6) Snatch High Pull: (75%/4)5   20:131:386
7) Press: (X/5)5   25:156:411

Day 4—Thursday (78 repetitions)
AM
1) Back Squat: 60%/2, 70%/2, (75%/5)4   24:24:435
2) Power Snatch: 60%/2, 65%/2, (70%/2)4   12:36:447
3) Power Clean & Jerk: 60%/2+2, 65%/2+2, (70%/2+2)4   24:60:471
4) Good Morning: (X/5)4   20:80:491

Day 5—Friday (135 repetitions)
AM
1) Front Squat: 60%/2, 70%/2, (75%/4)6   30:30:521
2) Clean High Pull: (80%/4)5   20:50:541
3) Push Press: 60%/4, 65%/4, (70%/3)5   23:73:564

PM
4) Snatch: 60%/3, 70%/3, (80%/3)3   15:88:579
5) Clean & Jerk: 60%/3+1, 70%/3+1, (80%/3+1)3   20:108:599
6) Back Squats: 60%/3, 70%/3, (80%/3)3   15:123:614
7) Press: (X/3)4   12:135:626

Day 6—Saturday (78 repetitions)
AM
1) Back Squat: 60%/2, 70%/2, (80%/3)4   16:16:642
2) Power Snatch: 60%/4, 65%/4, (70%/3)4   20:36:662
3) Power Clean & Jerk: 60%/4+2, 65%/4+2, (70%/3+2)3   27:63:689
4) Good Morning: (X/5)4   20:83:709

Day 7—Sunday
Rest

Week 2 (Preparation mesocycle) 542 repetitions

Day 8—Monday (141 repetitions)
AM
1) Back Squat: 60%/5, 70%/5, (75%/5)2, (80%/4)2   28:28:28
2) Snatch High Pull off blocks: (90%/5)4   20:48:48
3) Clean Deadlift: (95%/4)4   16:64:64

PM
4) Snatch:60%/3, 70%/3, (80%/3)5   21:85:85
5) Clean & Jerk: 60%/3+1, 70%/3+1, (80%/3+1)4   24:109:109
6) Push Press: 60%/4, 65%/4, (70%/3)4   20:129:129
7) Good Morning: (X/5)4   20:149:149

Day 9—Tuesday (60 repetitions)
AM
1) Back Squat: 60%/3, 70%/3, (80%/3)3   15:15:164
2) Power Snatch: 60%/4, 65%/4, (70%/4)3   20:35:184
3) Power Clean: 60%/4, 65%/4, (70%/4)3   20:55:204

Day 10—Wednesday (119 repetitions)
AM

1) Front Squat: 60%/4, 70%/4, (75%/4)2, (80%/4)2	24:24:228
2) Clean Extension: (80%/5)4	20:44:248
3) Behind the Neck Power Jerk: 60%/4, 65%/4, (70%/4)3	20:64:268

PM

4) Snatch: 60%/2, 70%/2, 80%/2, (85%/2)3	12:76:280
5) Clean & Jerk: 60%/2+2, 70%/2+2, 80%/2+2, (85%/2+2)3	24:100:304
6) Press: (X/5)4	20:120:324

Day 11—Thursday (60 repetitions)
AM

1) Back Squat: 60%/3, 70%/3, (80%/3)2, (85%/2)2	16:16:340
2) Power Snatch: 60%/4, 65%/4, (70%/4)3	20:36:360
3) Power Clean & Power Jerk: 60%/4+1, 65%/4+1, (70%/4+1)3	25:61:385

Day 12—Friday (103 repetitions)
AM

1) Back Squat: 60%/4, 70%/4, (80%/4)3	20:20:405
2) Snatch Deadlift: (105%/4)5	20:40:425
3) Behind the Neck Push Press: 60%/3, 65%/3, (70%/3)2	12:52:437

PM

4) Snatch High Pull and Snatch: 60%/3+1, 70%/3+1, (80%/3+1)3	20:72:457
5) Clean High Pull and Clean: 60%/3+1, 70%/3+1, (80%/3+1)3	20:92:477
6) Press: (X/3)4	12:104:489

Day 13—Saturday (60 repetitions)
AM

1) Back Squat: 60%/2, 70%/2, (80%/2)4	12:12:501
2) Power Snatch & Overhead Squat: 60%/3+3, 65%/3+3, (70%/3+3)2	24:36:525
3) Power Clean & Power Jerk: 60%/3+3, 65%/3+3, (70%/3+3)2	24:60:549

Day 14—Sunday
Rest

Week 3 (Preparation mesocycle) 637 repetitions

Day 15—Monday (166 repetitions)
AM

1) Back Squat: 60%/4, 70%/4, (80%/4)5	35:35:35
2) Clean High Pull: (80%/3)6	18:53:53
3) Behind the Neck Push Press: 60%/4, 65%/4, (70%/4)4	24:77:77

PM

4) Snatch: 60%/4, 70%/4, (80%/4)3	20:97:97
5) Clean & Jerk: 60%/4+1, 70%/4+1, (80%/4+1)3	25:122:122
6) Snatch Deadlift: (100%/2)5	10:132:132
7) Good Morning: (X/8)4	32:164:164

Day 16—Tuesday (70 repetitions)
AM

1) Back Squat: 60%/3, 70%/3, (80%/3)3	15:15:179
2) Power Snatch & Behind the Neck Push Press & Overhead Squat:	
60%/3+3+3, 65%/3+3+3, (70%/3+3+3)3	45:60:224
3) Power Clean: 60%/2, 65%/2, (70%/2)3	10:70:234

Day 17—Wednesday (121 repetitions)
AM

1) Front Squat: 60%/4, 70%/4, (80%/4)3	20:20:254
2) Snatch Extension: (85%/4)5	20:40:274
3) Power Jerk: 60%/3, 65%/3, (70%/3)4	18:58:292

PM

4) Snatch: 60%/2, 70%/2, (80%/2)2, (85%/2)2	12:70:304
5) Clean & Jerk: 60%/2+2, 70%/2+2, (80%/2+2)2, (85%/2+1)2	22:92:326
6) Clean High Pull: (80%/4)5	20:112:346
7) Press: (X/3)4	12:123:358

Day 18—Thursday (70 repetitions)
AM

1) Back Squat: 60%/2, 70%/2, (80%/2)6	16:16:374
2) Power Snatch: 60%/2, 65%/2, (70%/2)4	12:28:386
3) Power Clean & Front Squat & Jerk:	
60%/3+3+3, 65%/3+3+3, (70%/3+3+3)3	45:73:431

Day 19—Friday (140 repetitions)
AM

1) Back Squat: 60%/2, 70%/2, (80%/4)5	24:24:455
2) Clean Extension: (85%/4)5	20:44:475
3) Push Press: 60%/4, 65%/4, (70%/3)4	20:64:495

PM

4) Snatch: 60%/3, 70%/3, 80%/3, 85%/2, 80%/3, 85%/1	15:79:510
5) Clean & Jerk: 60%/2+3, 70%/2+3, 80%/3+2, 85%/2+1,	
80%/3+1, 85%/1+1	24:103:534
6) Snatch Extension: (95%/4)5	20:123:554
7) Press: (X/4)4	16:139:570

Day 20—Saturday (70 repetitions)
AM
1) Back Squat: 60%/2, 70%/2, (80%/2)4   12:12:582
2) Hang Power Snatch: 60%/2, 65%/2, (70%/2)4   12:24:594
3) Hang Power Clean: 60%/2, 65%/2, (70%/2)4   12:36:606
4) Snatch Deadlift on blocks: (90%/4)5   20:56:626
5) Press: (X/3)4   12:68:638

Week 4 (Preparation Mesocycle) 472 repetitions

Day 22—Monday (123 repetitions)
AM
1) Back Squat: (80%/4)5   20:20:20
2) Snatch High Pull: (85%/4)5   20:40:40
3) Push Press: 60%/4, 65%/4, (70%/4)4   24:64:64

PM
4) Snatch: (80%/4)5   20:84:84
5) Clean & Jerk: (80%/4+1)4   20:104:104
6) Clean Deadlift: (95%/3)6   18:122:122

Day 23—Tuesday (90 repetitions)
AM
1) Back Squat: (80%/3)5   15:15:137
2) Power Snatch & Behind the Neck Push Press & Overhead Squat:
     (70%/4+4+4)4   48:63:185
3) Clean Extension: 80%/4, (90%/4)5   24:87:209

Day 24—Wednesday (52 repetitions)
AM
1) Front Squat: (80%/4)5   20:20:229
2) Snatch: 60%/2, 70%/2, (80%/2)6   16:36:245
3) Clean & Jerk: 60%/2+1, 70%/2+1, (80%/2+1)6   24:60:269

Day 25—Thursday (104 repetitions)
AM
1) Back Squat: (80%/3)4   12:12:281
2) Power Snatch: 60%/3, 65%/3, (70%/3)4   18:30:299
3) Power Clean & Front Squat and Jerk: (70%/4+4+4)4   48:78:347

PM
4) Snatch Extension: (90%/4)5   20:98:367
5) Press: (X/3)4   12:110:379

Day 26—Friday (52 repetitions)
AM
1) Back Squat: (80%/4)5   20:20:399
2) Snatch: (80%/4)4   16:36:415
3) Clean & Jerk: (80%/4+1)3   15:51:430

Day 27—Saturday (52 repetitions)
AM
1) Back Squat: (80%/2)4   08:08:438
2) Hang Power Snatch: 60%/3, 65%/3, (70%/3)4   18:26:456
3) Hang Power Clean: 60%/3, 65%/3, (70%/3)4   18:44:474
4) Press: (X/3)4   12:56:486

Week 5—(Preparation Mesocycle) 708 repetitions

Day 29—Monday (184 repetitions)
AM
1) Back Squat: (80%/5)5   25:25:25
2) Clean Extensions: (90%/4)5   20:45:45
3) Snatch Deadlift: (105%/4)5   20:65:65
4) Press: (X/5)4   20:85:85

PM
5) Snatch: (80%/3)6   18:103:103
6) Clean & Jerk: (80%/3+1)6   24:127:127
7) Behind the Neck Push Press: 60%/5, 65%/5, (70%/4)4   26:153:153
8) Good Morning: (X/8)4   32:185:185

Day 30—Tuesday (78 repetitions)
AM
1) Back Squat: (80%3/, 85%/1)5   20:20:205
2) Power Snatch & Behind the Neck Push Press & Overhead Squat:
       (70%/4+4+4)4   48:68:253
3) Press: (X/3)4   12:80:265

Day 31—Wednesday (156 repetitions)
AM
1) Front Squat: (80%/5)5   25:25:290
2) Snatch Extension: (95%/4)5   20:45:310
3) Push Press: 60%/4, 65%/4, (70%/4)2   16:61:326

PM
4) Snatch: 60%/3, 70%/3, (80%/3, 85%/1)4   22:83:348
5) Clean & Jerk: 60%/3+2, 70%/3+2, (80%/3+1, 85%/1+1)4   36:119:384
6) Romanian Deadlift: (90%/5)5   25:144:409
7) Press: (X/3)4   12:156:421

Day 32—Thursday (78 repetitions)
AM
1) Back Squat: 60%/3, 70%/3, (80%/3)4   18:18:439
2) Power Clean & Front Squat & Jerk: (70%/4+4+4)4   48:66:487
3) Clean Extension: (85%/3)4   12:78:499

Day 33—Friday (135 repetitions)
AM
1) Back Squat: (80%/3)2, (85%/3)3   15:15:514
2) Snatch High Pull: (95%/4)6   24:39:538
3) Halting Clean Deadlift with 2 Halts: (80%/3)5   15:54:553

PM
4) Snatch: (80%/3, 85%/1)4   20:74:573
5) Clean & Jerk: (80%/3+1, 85%/1+2)4   28:102:601
6) Good Morning: (X/8)4   32:134:633

Day 34—Saturday (78 repetitions)
AM
1) Back Squat: (80%/3)6   18:18:651
2) Snatch Deadlift (up slow in 10 seconds) (80%/3)6   18:36:669
3) Romanian Deadlift: (90%/5)5   25:61:694
4) Push Press: 60%/4, 65%/4, (70%/4)3   20:81:714

Week 6 (Preparation Mesocycle) 637 repetitions

Day 36—Monday (166 repetitions)
AM
1) Back Squat: (80%/5)6   30:30:30
2) Snatch Exensions: (95%/4)6   24:54:54
3) Push Press: 60%/4, 65%/4, (70%/4)4   24:78:78

PM
4) Snatch: (80%/4)6   24:102:102
5) Clean & Jerk: (80%/4+1)5   25:127:127
6) Romanian Deadlift: (90%/5)6   30:157:157
7) Press: (X/3)4   12:169:169

Day 37—Tuesday (70 repetitions)
AM
1) Back Squat: (80%/3, 85%/2)6   25:25:194
2) Power Snatch & Behind the Neck Push Press & Overhead Squat:
        (70%/4+4+4)4   48:73:242

Day 38—Wednesday (140 repetitions)
AM
1) Front Squat: (80%/5)6   30:30:272
2) Clean Extensions: (90%/4)6   24:54:296
3) Jerk Behind Neck: (80%/4)5   20:74:316

PM
4) Snatch: 60%/3, 70%/3, (80%/3)6   24:98:340
5) Clean & Jerk: 60%/3+1, 70%/3+1, (80%/3+1)6   32:130:372
6) Snatch Extension: (105%/2)5   10:140:382

Day 39—Thursday (70 repetitions)
AM
1) Back Squat: (80%/3)6   18:18:400
2) Power Clean & Front Squat & Jerk: (70%/4+4+4)4   48:66:448

Day 40—Friday (121 repetitions)
AM
1) Back Squat: (85%/2)6   12:12:460
2) Snatch High Pull: (100%/3)8   24:36:484
3) Behind the Neck Power Jerk: 60%/3, 65%/3, 70%/3, (75%/3)4   21:57:505

PM
4) Snatch High Pull & Snatch: (80%/3+1)6   24:81:529
5) Clean High Pull & Clean: (80%/3+1)6   24:105:553
6) Good Morning: (X/6)4   24:129:577

Day 41—Saturday (70 repetitions)
AM
1) Back Squat: (85%/3)4   12:12:589
2) Power Snatch: 60%/2, 65%/2, 70%/2, (75%/2)3   12:24:601
3) Power Clean: 60%/2, 65%/2, 70%/2, (75%/2)3   12:36:613
4) Push Press: 60%/3, 65%/3, (70%/3)5   21:47:634

Week 7 (Preparation Mesocycle) 472 Repetitions

Day 43—Monday (123 repetitions)
AM
1) Back Squat: (80%/5)3, (85%/3)3   24:24:24
2) Halting Clean Deadlift with 2 halts: (80%/3)6   18:42:42
3) Snatch Extension: (100%/3)6   18:60:60

PM
4) Snatch: (85%/3)6   18:78:78
5) Clean & Jerk: (85%/3+1)5   20:98:98
6) Good Morning: (X/6)4   24:122:122

Day 44—Tuesday (104 repetitions)
AM
1) Back Squat: (80%/3)6   18:18:140
2) Snatch Deadlift: (105%/3)6   18:36:158
3) Press: (X/4)5   20:56:178

PM
4) Power Snatch: 60%/4, 65%/4, (70%/4)4   24:80:202
5) Power Clean: 60%/4, 65%/4, (70%/4)4   24:104:226

Day 45—Wednesday (52 repetitions)
AM
1) Front Squat: (85%/3)6   18:18:244
2) Snatch: (85%/2)8   16:34:260
3) Clean & Jerk: (85%/2+1)7   21:55:281

Day 46—Thursday (90 repetitions)
AM
1) Back Squat: (80%/3)5   15:15:296
2) Snatch: (80%/2)6   12:27:308
3) Clean & Jerk: (80%/2+1)6   18:45:326
4) Snatch Extension: (105%/3)5   15:60:341
5) Clean Deadlift: (95%/3)5   15:75:356
6) Press: (X/3)5   15:90:371

Day 47—Friday (52 repetitions)
AM
1) Back Squat: (85%/2)5   10:10:381
2) Power Snatch: 60%/3, 65%/3, 70%/3, (75%/2)4   17:27:398
3) Power Clean & Jerk: 60%/3+1, 65%/3+1, 70%/3+1, (75%/2+1)4   24:51:422

Day 48—Saturday (52 repetitions)
AM
1) Back Squat: (80%/4)4   16:16:438
2) Snatch: (80%/2)5   10:26:448
3) Clean & Jerk: (80%/2+2)5   20:46:468
4) Press: (X/2)4   08:54:476

Week 8 (Preparation mesocycle) 542 repetitions

Day 50—Monday (141 repetitions)
AM
1) Back Squat: (80%/5)3, (85%/3)3   24:24:24
2) Halting Snatch Deadlift with 2 Halts: (80%/3)6   18:42:42
3) Clean Extension: (90%/3)5   15:57:57
4) Push Press: 60%/4, 65%/4, (70%/4)5   28:85:85

PM
5) Snatch: (80%/2)3, (85%/2)3   12:97:97
6) Clean & Jerk: (80%/2+1)3, (85%/2+1)3   18:115:115
7) Good Morning: (X/6)4   24:139:139

Day 51--Tuesday (60 repetitions)
AM
1) Back Squat: (80%/3)5   15:15:154
2) Snatch: 60%/2, 70%/2, (80%/2)6   16:31:170
3) Clean & Jerk: 60%/2+1, 70%/2+1, (80%/2+1)5   21:52:191
4) Behind the Neck Power Jerk: 60%/2, 70%/2, (75%/2)3   10:62:201

Day 52—Wednesday (119 repetitions)
AM
1) Front Squat: (80%/5, 85%/2)5   35:35:236
2) Snatch Extension: (90%/5)5   25:60:261
3) Clean Halting Deadlift with 2 Halts (80%/3)5   15:75:276

PM
4) Snatch: (80%/3, 90%/1)4   16:91:292
5) Clean & Jerk: (80%/3+1, 90%/1+1)4   24:115:316

Day 53--Thursday (60 repetitions)
AM
1) Back Squat: (80%/3)5   15:15:331
2) Power Snatch: 60%/3, 65%/3, (70%/3)2, (75%/2)2   16:31:347
3) Power Clean & Power Jerk: 60%/3+2, 65%/3+2,
       (70%/3+2)2, (75%/2+2)2   28:59:375

Day 54--Friday (103 repetitions)
AM
1) Back Squat: (80%/3, 85%/1)4   16:16:391
2) Clean High Pull: (80%/4)6   24:40:415
3) Push Press: 60%/4, 65%/4, (70%/4)4   24:64:439

PM
4) Snatch: (80%/3)4   12:76:451
5) Clean & Jerk: (80%/3+1)4   16:92:467
6) Press: (X/3)4   12:104:479

Day 55--Saturday (60 repetitions)
AM
1) Back Squat: (80%/2)6   12:12:491
2) Power Snatch:60%/3, 65%/3, (70%/3)5   21:33:511
3) Power Clean & Power Jerk: 60%/3+2, 65%/3+2, (70%/3+2)4   30:63:541

Week 9 (Preparation Mesocycle) 708 Repetitions

Day 57—Monday (184 repetitions)
AM
1) Back Squat: (85%/4)5   20:20:20
2) Snatch Extension: (100%/3)6   18:38:38
3) Clean Deadlift (95%/3)5   15:53:53
4) Push Press: 60%/4, 65%/4, (70%/4)5   28:81:81

PM
5) Snatch: (80%/4)6   24:105:105
6) Clean & Jerk: (80%/4+1)6   30:135:135
7) Back Squat: (80%/2)5   10:145:145
8) Behind the Neck Power Jerk: (70%/3)3, (80%/3)3   18:163:163
9) Good Morning: (X/5)4   20:183:183

Day 58—Tuesday (78 repetitions)
AM
1) Back Squat: 60%/2, 70%/2, (80%/2)4   12:12:195
2) Snatch: 60%/2, 70%/2, (80%/2)4   12:24:207
3) Clean & Jerk: 60%/2+1, 70%/2+1, (80%/2+1)4   18:42:225
4) Snatch Deadlift: (105%/3)5   15:57:240
5) Press: (X/4)5   20:77:260

Day 59—Wednesday (156 repetitions)
AM
1) Front Squat: (85%/4)5   20:20:280
2) Power Snatch: 60%/2, 65%/2, (70%/4)5   24:44:304
3) Power Clean & Power Jerk: 60%/2+2, 65%/2+2, (70%/4+2)5   38:82:342

PM
4) Clean Extension: (95%/3)5   15:97:357
5) Hang Snatch High Pulls from below Knees: (80%/4)5   20:117:377
6) Push Press: 60%/4, 65%/4, (70%/4)4   24:141:401
7) Good Morning: (X/4)4   16:157:417

Day 60—Thursday (78 repetitions)
AM
1) Back Squat: (80%/2)5   10:10:427
2) Snatch: 60%/2, 70%/2, (80%/2)2, (85%/2)2   12:22:439
3) Clean & Jerk: 60%/2+2, 70%/2+2, (80%/2+2)2, (85%/2+2)2   24:46:463
4) Romanian Deadlift: (95%/5)6   30:76:493

Day 61—Friday (135 repetitions)
AM
1) Back Squat: (80%/3)8   24:24:517
2) Snatch High Pull: (100%/3)6   18:42:535
3) Clean Deadlift: (85%/3)5   15:57:550
4) Behind the Neck Push Press: 60%/4, 65%/4, (70%/4, 75%/2)3   26:83:576

PM
5) Snatch: 60%/3, 70%/3, (80%/3)4   18:101:594
6) Clean: 60%/3, 70%/3, (80%/3)4   18:119:612
7) Press: (X/4)4   16:135:628

Day 62—Saturday (78 repetitions)
AM
1) Back Squat: 60%/2, 70%/2, (80%/2)6   16:16:644
2) Power Snatch: 60%/3, (70%/3)4   15:31:659
3) Power Clean: 60%/3, (70%/3)4   15:46:674
4) Clean Extension: (90%/3)6   18:64:692
5) Snatch Deadlift (105%/4)5   20:84:712

Week 10 (Preparation Mesocycle) 542 repetitions

Day 64—Monday (141 repetitions)
AM
1) Back Squat: (85%/4, 90%/1)5   25:25:25
2) Snatch High Pull: (105%/3)6   18:43:43
3) Clean Deadlift: (100%/4)5   20:63:63

PM
4) Snatch: 60%/1, 70%/1, 80%/1, 85%/1, 90%/1, (85%/3)4   17:80:80
5) Clean & Jerk: 60%/1+1, 70%/1+1, 80%/1+1, 85%/1+1,
      90%/1+1, (85%/3+1)4   26:106:106
6) Press: (X/4)4   16:122:122
7) Good Morning: (X/6)4   24:146:146

Day 65—Tuesday (60 repetitions)
AM
1) Back Squat: (80%/3)6   18:18:164
2) Snatch: (80%/2)6   12:30:176
3) Clean & Jerk: (80%/2+1)6   18:48:184
4) Power Jerk: 70%/3, (75%/3)2, (80%/3)2   15:63:199

Day 66—Wednesday (119 repetitions)
AM
1) Front Squat: (85%/4, 90%/1)5   25:25:224
2) Clean Extension: (95%/3)6   18:43:242
3) Behind the Neck Push Press: 60%/4, 65%/4, (70%/4)2, (75%/2)2   20:63:262

PM
4) Power Snatch: 60%/4, 65%/4, 70%/4, 75%/2, 70%/4, 75%/1   19:82:281
5) Power Clean & Power Jerk: 60%/4+2, 65%/4+1, 70%/4+1,
      75%/2+1, 70%/4+1, 75%/1+1   26:89:288
6) Snatch Extension: (100%/3)5   15:104:303
7) Power Jerk:(70%/3)3, (75%/3)3   18:122:321

Day 67—Thursday (60 repetitions)
AM
1) Back Squat: (85%/2)5   10:10:331
2) Snatch: (80%/3)4   12:22:343
3) Clean & Jerk: (80%/3+1)4   16:38:359
4) Clean Deadlift: (100%/3)4   12:50:371
5) Press: (X/3)4   12:62:383

Day 68—Friday (103 repetitions)
AM
1) Back Squat: (80%/3)4   12:12:395
2) Snatch High Pull: (95%/4)5   20:32:415
3) Push Press: 60%/3, 65%/3, (70%/3)2, (75%/3)2   18:50:433

PM
1) Power Snatch & Overhead Squat: 60%/2+3, (70%/2+3)2, (75%/2+3)2 25:75:458
2) Power Clean & Power Jerk: 60%/2+3, (70%/2+3)2, (75%/2+3)2   25:100:483

Day 69—Saturday (60 repetitions)
AM
1) Front Squat: (80%/3)5   15:15:498
2) Snatch: (80%/3, 85%/2)3   15:30:513
3) Clean & Jerk: (80%/3+1, 85%/2+1)3   21:51:534
4) Press: (X/3)4   12:63:546

Week 11 (Preparation Mesocycle) 637 repetitions

Day 71—Monday (166)
AM
1) Back Squat: (85%/4)6   24:24:24
2) Snatch High Pull: (105%/3)7   21:45:45
3) Clean Deadlift: (100%/4)6   24:69:69
4) Press: (X/2)4   08:77:77

PM
5) Snatch: 60%/2, 70%/2, 80%/2, (85%/3, 90%/1)5   26:103:103
6) Clean & Jerk: 60%/2+1, 70%/2+1, 80%/2+1, (85%/3+1, 90%/1+1)4   33:136:136
7) Good Morning: (X/8)432:168:168

Day72—Tuesday (70 repetitions)
AM
1) Back Squat: (85%/2)6   12:12:180
2) Snatch: (85%/2)6   12:24:192
3) Clean & Jerk: (85%/2+2)5   20:44:212
4) Clean Extension: (95%/3)6   18:62:230
5) Press: (X/2)4   08:70:238

Day 73—Wednesday (140 repetitions)
AM
1) Front Squat: (85%/4)6   24:24:262
2) Clean High Pull: (95%/3)6   18:42:280
3) Jerk off Rack: (80%/4)6   24:66:304

PM
4) Power Snatch: 60%/3, 65%/3, (70%/3)2, (75%/3)2   18:84:322
5) Power Clean & Jerk: 60%/3+1, 65%/3+1, (70%/3+1)2, (75%/3+1)2   24:108:346
6) Romanian Deadlift: (100%/5)6   30:138:376

Day 74—Thursday (70 repetitions)
AM
1) Back Squat: (80%/3)5   15:15:391
2) Snatch: (85%/2)6   12:24:403
3) Clean & Jerk: (85%/2+2)5   20:44:423
4) Push Press: 60%/2, (70%/2)3, (75%/2)3   14:58:435
5) Front Squat: (85%/2)6   12:70:447

Day 75—Friday (121 repetitions)
AM
1) Back Squat: (85%/3, 90%/2)6   30:30:477
2) Snatch Extension: (105%/2)8   16:46:483
3) Power Jerk: 60%/2, 70%/2, (75%/2, 80%/1)3   13:59:496

PM
4) Snatch: (80%/3)5   15:74:511
5) Clean & Jerk: (80%/3+1)5   20:94:531
6) Clean Halting Deadlift: (90%/4)6   24:118:555

Day 76—Saturday (70 repetitions)
AM
1) Front Squat: (80%/3)5   15:15:570
2) Power Snatch: 60%/2, 70%/2, (75%/2)4   12:27:582
3) Power Clean & Jerk: 60%/2+2, 70%/2+2, (75%/2+2)3   20:47:602
4) Snatch Extension: (95%/4)5   20:67:622
5) Press: (X/3)4   12:79:634

Week 12 (Preparation Mesocycle) 472 repetitions

Day 78—Monday (123 repetitions)
AM
1) Back Squat: (85%/3, 90%/2, 95%/1)5   30:30:30
2) Snatch High Pull: (105%/3)6   18:48:48
3) Push Press: 60%/2, (70%/3, 75%/1)4   18:66:66

PM
4) Snatch: (80%/3, 85%/2, 90%/1)4   24:90:90
5) Clean & Jerk: (80%/3+1, 85%/2+1, 90%/1+1)4   36:126:126

Day 79—Tuesday (90 repetitions)
AM
1) Back Squat: (85%/3)5   15:15:141
2) Snatch: (85%/2, 90%/1)5   15:30:156
3) Clean & Jerk: (85%/2+1, 90%/1+1)5   25:55:181
4) Clean Deadlift: (100%/3)5   15:70:196
5) Good Morning: (X/5)4   20:90:216

Day 80—Wednesday (52 repetitions)
AM
1) Front Squat: (85%/3, 90%/2, 95%/1)5   30:30:246
2) Power Snatch: 60%/2, (70%/2, 75%/2)4   18:48:264
3) Press: (X/2)4   08:56:272

Day 81—Thursday (104 repetitions)
AM
1) Back Squat: (85%/3, 90%/1)4   16:16:288
2) Clean Extension: (105%/2)5   10:26:298
3) Behind the Neck Power Jerk: 60%/3, 70%/3, (75%/3, 80%/1)3   18:44:316

PM
4) Snatch: (80%/3, 85%/2, 90%/1)5   30:74:346
5) Clean & Jerk: (80%/3+1, 85%/2+1, 90%/1+1)4   36:110:382

Day 82—Friday (52 repetitions)
AM
1) Back Squat: (85%/3)4   12:12:394
2) Power Snatch: 60%/2, 70%/2, (75%/2, 80%/1)3   13:25:407
3) Power Clean & Jerk: 60%/2+1, 70%/2+1, (75%/2+1, 80%/1+1)3   21:46:428
4) Press: (X/2)4   08:54:436

Day 83—Saturday (52 repetitions)
AM
1) Front Squat: (80%/4)3, (85%/3)3   21:21:457
2) Snatch: (80%/3, 85%/2, 90%/1)3   18:39:475
3) Clean & Jerk: (80%/3+1, 85%/1+1, 90%/1+1)2   20:59:495

Week 13 (Pre-Competition Mesocycle) 450 repetitions

Day 85—Monday (117 repetitions)
AM
1) Snatch: 60%/2, 70%/2, 80%/2, 85%/2, (90%/2)5   18:18:18
2) Clean & Jerk: 60%/2+1, 70%/2+1, 80%/2+1, 85%/2+1,
      (90%/2+1, 90%/1+1)3   27:45:45
3) Snatch High Pull: (95%/3)6   18:63:63

PM
4) Back Squat: 80%/3, (85%/3, 90%/2)4   23:86:86
5) Power Jerk: 60%/3, 70%/3, (75%/3, 80%/1)3   18:104:104
6) Clean Deadlift: (100%/2)6   12:116:116

Day 86—Tuesday (50 repetitions)
AM
1) Snatch: (85%/2)3, (90%/2)3   12:12:128
2) Clean & Jerk: (85%/2+1)3, (90%/2+1)2, 90%/1+1   17:29:157
3) Clean Extension: (95%/2)5   10:39:167
4) Press: (X/3)4 12:51:179

Day 87—Wednesday (99 repetitions)
AM
1) Power Snatch: 60%/3, (70%/3, 75%/2, 80%/1)3	21:21:200
2) Power Clean & Jerk: 60%/3+1, (70%/3+1, 75%/2+1, 80%/1+1)3	31:52:231
3) Snatch Extension: (105%/2)6	12:64:243
4) Front Squat: (80%/4)2, (85%/3, 90%/2, 95%/1)3	26:90:269
5) Push Press: 60%/2, 70%/2, (75%/2)2	08:98:277

Day 88—Thursday (50 repetitions)
AM
1) Snatch: 80%/3, 85%/2, 90%/2, 80%/2, 85%/2, 90%/1, (80%/3)3	21:21:298
2) Clean & Jerk: 80%/3+1, 85%/2+1, 90%/2+1, 80%/2+1, 85%/2+1, 90%/1+1, (80%/3+1)3	30:51:328

Day 89—Friday (86 repetitions)
AM
1) Power Snatch & Overhead Squat: 60%/3+4, (70%/2+3)2, (75%/2+3)2	27:27:355
2) Power Clean & Power Jerk: 60%/3+3, (70%/2+3)2, (75%/2+3)2	26:53:381
3) Clean Extension: 80%/3, 90%/3, (95%/2)4	14:67:395
4) Front Squat: 80%/1, 85%/1, 90%/1, (95%/1)5, (80%/3)4	20:87:415

Day 90—Saturday (50 repetitions)
AM
1) Snatch: (80%/3, 85%/2, 90%/2)3	21:21:436
2) Clean & Jerk: (80%/3+1, 85%/2+1, 90%/2+1)3	24:45:460

Week 14 (Pre-competition Mesocycle) 345 repetitions

Day 92—Monday (45 repetitions)
AM
1) Snatch: 60%/2, 70%/2, 80%/2, (85%/2, 90%/1)4	18:18:18
2) Clean & Jerk: 60%/2+1, 70%/2+1, 80%/2+1, (85%/2+1, 90%/1+1)3	24:42:42

Day 93—Tuesday (104 repetitions)
AM
1) Snatch: (85%/2)6	12:12:54
2) Clean & Jerk: (85%/2+1)5	15:27:69
3) Snatch High Pull: (100%/3)5	15:42:84
4) Back Squat: (85%/3, 90%/2, 95%/1)4	24:66:108

PM
5) Clean Deadlift: (100%/3)6	18:84:126
6) Power Jerk: 60%/3, (70%/3, 75%/2, 80%/1)3	21:105:147

Day 94—Wednesday
Rest

Day 95—Thursday (93 repetitions)
AM
1) Power Snatch: 65%/3, (70%/3, 75%/2, 80%/1)4   27:27:174
2) Power Clean & Jerk: 65%/3+1, (70%/3+1, 75%/2+1, 80%/1+1)4   40:67:214
3) Front Squat: (85%/3, 90%/2, 95%/1)4   24:91:238

Day 96—Friday (52 repetitions)
AM
1) Snatch: (85%/2, 90%/1)5   15:15:253
2) Clean & Jerk: (85%/2+1, 90%/1+1)5   25:40:278
3) Clean High Pull: (95%/3)4   12:52:290

Day 97—Saturday (52 repetitions)
AM
1) Snatch: 80%/1, 85%/1, (90%/1)3, (80%/3)3   14:14:304
2) Clean & Jerk: 80%/1+1, 85%/1+1, (90%/1+1)2, (80%/3+1)2   14:28:318
3) Back Squat: 80%/1, 85%/1, (90%/1)2, (95%/1)2 (80%/3)3   15:43:333
4) Press: (X/3)4 12:55:345

Week 15 (Pre-Competition Mesocycle) 405 Repetitions

Day 99—Monday (122 repetitions)
AM
1) Snatch: singles to max, (max-10, max-5, max)3   15:15:15
2) Clean & Jerk: singles to max, (max-10, max-5, max)3   30:45:45
3) Snatch Extension: (105%/3)4   12:57:57

PM
4) Front Squat: singles to max, (max-10, max-5, max)3   15:72:72
5) Power Jerk: 60%/2, 70%/2, (80%/2)4   12:84:84
6) Clean Extension: (95%/2)5   10:94:94
7) Press: (X/3)4   12:106:106
8) Good Morning: (X/4)4   16:122:122

Day 100—Tuesday (61 repetitions)
AM
1) Snatch: 60%/2, 70%/2, 80%/2, (85%/2, 90%/1)3   15:15:137
2) Clean & Jerk: 60%/2+1, 70%/2+1, 80%/2+1, (85%/2+1, 90%/1+1)3   24:39:161
3) Snatch High Pull: (95%/2)5   10:49:171
4) Push Press: (70%/3)4   12:61:183

Day 101—Wednesday (0 repetitions)
Rest

Day 102—Thursay (109 repetitions)
AM
1) Power Snatch: singles to max, (max-10, max-5, max)3   13:13:192
2) Power Clean & Jerk: singles to max, (max-10, max-5, max)3   26:39:222
3) Clean Extension: (90%/3, 95%/2)3   15:54:237

PM
4) Back Squat: singles to max (max-10, max-5, max)3   15:69:252
5) Snatch Extension: (105%/2)6   12:81:264
6) Clean Deadlift: (100%/3)4   12:93:276
7) Press: (X/3)5   15:108:291

Day 103—Friday (53 repetitions)
AM
1) Snatch: singles to max, (max-10, max-5, max)3   15:15:304
2) Clean & Jerk: singles to max, (max-10, max-5, max)3   30:45:334
3) Clean Extension: (100%/2)4   08:53:342

Day 104—Saturday (61 repetitions)
AM
1) Power Snatch: 60%/2, 65%/2, (70%/2)4   12:12:354
2) Power Clean & Jerk: 60%/2+1, 65%/2+1, (70%/2+1)4   18:30:372
3) Front Squat: 60%/3, 70%/3, 80%/3, (85%/3)4   21:51:393
4) Press: (X/2)5   10:61:403

Week 16 (Pre-Competition Mesocycle) 300 repetitions

Day 106—Monday (105 repetitions)
AM
1) Snatch: singles to max, (max-10, max-5, max)2   12:12:12
2) Clean & Jerk: singles to max, (max-10, max-5, max)2   24:36:36
3) Snatch Extension: (105%/2)6   12:48:48

PM
4) Front Squat: singles to max, (max-10, max-5, max)2   12:60:60
5) Clean Deadlift: (105%/3)4   12:72:72
6) Jerk off Rack: (80%/3)2, (85%/2)2, 90%/1, 80%/3, 85%/2, 90%/1   17:89:89
7) Good Morning: (X/5)4   20:109:109

Day 107—Tuesday (45 repetitions)
AM
1) Snatch: (85%/2)5   10:10:119
2) Clean & Jerk: (85%/2+1)4   12:22:131
3) Clean Extension: (95%/2)5   10:32:141
4) Press: (X/3)4   12:44:153

Day 108—Wednesday
Rest

Day 109—Thursday (84 repetitions)
AM
1) Snatch: singles to max, (max-10, max-5, max)2	12:12:165
2) Clean & Jerk: singles to max, (max-10, max-5, max)2	24:36:189
3) Back Squat: singles to max, (max-10, max-5, max)2	12:48:201
4) Snatch High Pull: (95%/3)5	15:63:216
5) Jerk off rack: (80%/3, 85%/2, 90%/1, 95%/1)3	21:84:237

Day 110—Friday
Rest

Day 111—Friday (66 repetitions)
AM
1) Power Snatch: singles to max, (max-10, max-5, max)2	10:10:247
2) Power Clean & Jerk: singles to max, (max-10, max-5, max)2	20:30:267
3) Front Squat: (80%/3, 85%/3, 90%/1, 95%/1)2	16:46:283
4) Clean Extension: (90%/2)4	08:54:291
5) Press: (X/3)4	12:66:303

Week 17 (Pre-competition Mesocycle) 150 repetitions

Day 113—Monday (63 repetitions)
AM
1) Snatch: 60%/1, 70%/1, 80%/1, (85%/1, 90%/1, 95%/1)3	12:12:12
2) Clean & Jerk: 60%/1+1, 70%/1+1, 80%/1+1,	
(85%/1+1, 90%/1+1, 95%/1+1)3	24:36:36
3) Front Squat: 80%/3, 85%/2, 90%/1, 95%/1, 80%/3, 85%/2, 90%/1	13:49:49
4) Snatch Extension: (85%/2)5	10:59:59
5) Press: (X/2)4	08:67:67

Day 114—Tuesday (39 repetitions)
AM
1) Power Snatch: (60%/1, 70%/1, 75%/1)3	09:09:76
2) Power Clean & Jerk: (60%/1+1, 70%/1+1, (75%/1+1)3	18:27:94
3) Back Squat: 60%/2, 70%/2, (80%/2)2, (85%/2)2	12:39:106

Day 115—Wednesday
Rest

Day 116—Thursday (48 repetitions)
1) Snatch: 60%/1, 70%/1, (80%/1, 85%/1, 90%/1)2	08:08:114
2) Clean & Jerk: 60%/1+1, 70%/1+1, (80%/1+1, 85%/1+1, 90%/1+1)2	16:24:130
3) Jumping Back Squat: (50%/3)4	12:36:142
4) Press: (X/3)4	12:48:154

Day117—Friday
Rest

Day 118—Saturday
Rest

Day 119—Sunday
Competition

SECTION E
RESTORATION

Restoration is a process that normally takes place when the physiology of the body is disrupted. For very young athletes or non-athletes, the body restores itself to its normal level of functioning from day to day. This is a typical homeostatic activity. When the extent of the disruption (stress) becomes greater and exceeds the restorative capabilities of the organism, there is a temporary disruption of activity.

Talented athletes who have undergone GPP during the optimal window of time can withstand greater levels of stress before the normal activity levels are disrupted. Well-planned and implemented GPP increases local circulation, improves the functioning of the endocrines and the capacity of the lungs for gas exchange. All three of these factors are especially valuable for the restoration process.

Another function that is frequently overlooked is the efficiency of the digestive system in the processes of chemical breakdown and absorption. A healthful regimen of appropriate diet and physical activity will lead to digestive efficiency during the pubertal and adolescent stages.

The function of a restoration regime is to increase the capacity of the organism to withstand greater and more frequent training loads.

What takes place during restoration is an elimination of metabolites from the affected tissues, an increase in the movement of molecules at the local levels and subsequently an increased collision rate that will result in chemical activity to form new molecules or breakdown existing ones. To accomplish these tasks, the delivery of substances must be heightened through increased circulation.

The most effective restoration will take place with the least amount of caloric expenditure on the part of the organism. The restoration activities must be undertaken in a passive manner.

There are several modalities available for the restoration process, and like any stimulus, there is an adaptive response that will eventually minimize the effects of the stimulus. Because of this adaptation, the modalities must be regularly rotated in order to have a continued effect on the organism.

While coaches and sports administrators spend a considerable amount of effort attempting to learn and implement the most effective training programs, restoration is largely ignored, although its importance in the development of the athletes increases as the athlete progresses toward higher levels of sports achievement.

An effective restoration program will allow the athlete to maintain greater training loads on more consecutive days of training. This will have the long-term effect of increasing the annual training load.

Whereas athlete A might be able to maintain a great training volume for two consecutive days, athlete B with superior restoration might be able to maintain that load for a another day. This could result in many more days of heavier loads over the course of the year, and hence a significantly improved level of performance.

With the most effective anti-doping technology in place for the top Olympic athletes on the planet, illicit Performance Enhancing Drugs (PED) will become less and less of a factor in athletic development. Conversely, restoration will grow to be of greater and greater importance.

Just a brief comment on the Performance Enhancing Drug issue from the standpoint of a coach who has had to deal with the issue for years. Both the drug dealers and the drug cops (WADA) have some interest in maintaining the mythology of performance enhancing drugs. Drug providers are hyping their product and they have a great deal to gain by convincing athletes that drugs can transform a mediocre athlete into a world-beater.

WADA receives funding from a variety of sources to go after drug takers. If they effectively do their job, they eliminate the necessity for their existence. If athletes are convinced that there are minimal benefits to drug usage that are not worth the risk of detection, they are less apt to use drugs and lessen the necessity for drug testing.

If properly applied restoration completely eclipsed any PED usage, both groups would be out of business. And since neither group derives any income from restoration services or technology, they have no interest in promoting restoration as an alternative means of improving athletic performance.

Due to the lack of demand there has not been a great deal of effort put into the development of more effective restoration technologies. We are quite possibly now at the dawn of enhanced restoration, and those nations interested in attaining the best outcomes internationally will pursue the development of those enhanced technologies with vigor.

CHAPTER 15
RESTORATIVE MEANS

Restoration is the process is returning the muscles, endocrines and other associated tissues and organ to a normal resting state between training sessions. It consists of breaking down accumulated metabolites within the muscles and inducing greater circulation in order to remove those molecules and to replace them with nutrients that will aid the tissues in recovery. It also involves the secretion of anabolic hormones and increasing those hormones' capacities to access the cells. It also aids in improving lymphodrainage. The means by which these processes can be facilitated are several and varied.

Although I have extensive experience in training weightlifters, I have never had the necessary access to sufficient restoration modalities to fully explore the possibilities and become expert in managing their implementation. I have, however, had considerable experience with athletes who were able to make some regular use of some of them and found that it greatly enhanced their capacities to train with greater intensities, higher loads and greater frequencies.

I've found it rather odd, naïve or ignorant that the U.S. Olympic Training Center has been rather lax in dealing with the issue of restoration for weightlifters and other athletes housed at the Colorado Springs facility. During those periods when I served as a coach for the weightlifting program, there was always some resistance to the provision of restoration facilities and therapists.

Since the use of pharmacology falls within the category of restoration, and the USOC was justifiably taking such a staunch position against the use of performance enhancing drugs, it would only seem reasonable to expect them to emphasize other modalities of restoration in order to minimize the necessity to employ pharmaceuticals. This was never the case. I would expect an NOC to take the lead in providing the best means of restoration for athletes in hard training. The USOC has for years chosen to minimize if not ignore the issue or merely give it lip service. If the goal of USOC is to win medals at the Olympics and Pan American Games, then any legal means of increasing the ability to train effectively would have to be a priority item.

It is well known that the restoration rate after stressful exercise is a key factor in maintaining progress in athletic conditioning. The capacity of the body to restore itself is in direct relationship to the metabolic rate, and thus athletic development takes place most rapidly in young, mature adults and in weightlifters in the lower bodyweight classes. As an athlete gains weight and/or ages, restoration becomes a more important factor in the enabling of increased training loads.

The first factor to be considered by the coach is the talent of the athlete. There is such a thing as metabolic talent, and the top athletes have the capacity to restore at a much higher rate than the average person. Generally, high energy levels during youth are good indicators of high restoration rate. They are reflective of good circulation and exchange rates of materials in the body.

The second factor is the appropriate use of general physical preparation before and during adolescence to enhance the circulatory machinery of the body and the development of receptor sites for those molecules that will influence the restorative processes at the cellular and subcellular levels.

The proper application of restorative means in the developmental training process will allow greater and greater training loads to be imposed on the athlete. During the stages of the mature athlete's career, restoration is absolutely necessary to maintain continued progress.

Restorative means must be varied in order to remain effective, as the body can adapt to the various restoration modalities. It is best conducted in a restoration facility located near the training facilities that has the various modalities conveniently available. Restoration should, above all, not require an inordinate energy expenditure, as that would undermine a major purpose for which it is employed. The inclusion of restoration sessions in the daily regimen goes hand in hand with the planning and organization of feeding, sleeping and training in the organization of the daily regimen. As the weightlifter proceeds through a career, the greater the need for a well-structured daily regimen will be. As the results grow, the proper timing and implementation of feeding, sleeping and restoration become much more critical, and hence the greater the need for more rigidity in the daily schedule.

Table 15.1 reflects a restoration regimen for an athlete in serious training. It was originally presented in *Secrets of Soviet Sports Fitness and Training* by Yessis and Trubo. Dr. Yessis was a serious student of Soviet training methods and was able to obtain this information during visits to the Soviet Union during the heyday of Soviet sports.

Table 15.1 illustrates how there is a regular cycling of restoration modalities throughout the week. The reason that the modalities are varied with regularity is that the body adapts to one or two modalities over time and they lose their effectiveness. In order to prevent this from occurring a system of rotation must be instituted.

Pedagogical Means

Restoration can be enhanced through the psychological approach of the athlete toward the individual training session and the long-term training plan. The coach must also be involved in some of these decisions and processes.

The structure of the individual session as far as warm-up, exercise selection, exercise order, loading, cool down and rest periods between sets can be modified so that the session is most productive and leads to a subsequent equally productive session. Since each rest period between sets is a form of restoration, the athlete must be sure to pace the training in a manner that allows for sufficient restoration between sets. A training session performed with insufficient rest between sets will affect the capacity to train the next day.

On a more long-term basis, the more advanced lifters will have to communicate information about restfulness of sleep, appetite and other non-training factors in order that the training can be appropriately modified to achieve the desired goals of each mesocycle and macrocycle. This skillful manipulation of the training is part of the art of coaching

Training Load and Means of Restoration (in minutes)	Days of the Week							Weekly Total
	1	2	3	4	5	6	7	
Morning	45	45	45	45	45	45	45	315
Daytime	150	90	120		150	90		600
Evening	90		90		90	90		360
General Physical Preparation	30	60	30	90	30	60	60	360
Total For The Day	315	195	285	135	315	285	105	1635
Means of Restoration								
hand massage		30				30		60
vibrational massage	15		30		20			65
"electrical" vibro-bath		20						20
contrast baths		5				5		10
water showers	10	5	10	10	10	5	10	60
Sharko shower		5				5		10
flowing stream shower		5				5		10
ultraviolet irradiation		5		5		5		15
heat bath (sauna)		15				15		30
pine neeedle baths	10			10				20
psychorehabilitation	30					30		60
Total For The Day	65	90	40	25	30	100	10	360

Table 15.1 Training Loads and Restoration Means. Note: A Sharko shower is a high pressure shower (1.5 atmospheres) at 15--20°C from a distance of 3.5 meters.

and one of the key reasons for the failure of "train you by mail" approaches.

Of course it requires that a coach be working with a manageable number of athletes in order to keep track of all the details surrounding each athlete's case. On my study tour of Bulgaria, I was informed that the top professional coaches were responsible for no more than four athletes each.

Common Means and Local Means

Restoration means can be divided into two broad categories. Common Means are more general and include full body massage, UV light, ionization and various forms of hydrotherapy. Local Means include local body massage, electrostimulation and ultrasound. The first category is best applied after periods of great training, while the second works best after individual training sessions. If the athlete is training multiple sessions per day, local means should be employed after individual sessions, but common means at the end of the day.

Balneology

Balneology is the process of stimulating circulation through immersion of the body in mineral salt and aromatic baths. The effervescence of the solution along with the heat and the hydrostatic pressure significantly increases general circulation. The use of a Jacuzzi can also increase the frictional resistance and hence the therapeutic value of warm water immersion. This increased blood flow has the dual purpose of providing greater availability of oxygen, macro- and micro-nutrients and hormones, while removing metabolites from the distressed tissue and increasing lymphodrainage. The regular use of hot mineral baths has long been a staple of many health spas, but it has a definite role in the restoration of hard training athletes.

The temperature should be at approximately 35°C, and the time of immersion for weightlifters should be between 12 and 15 minutes. Some guidelines for water temperatures are shown in Table 15.2.

Very cold	10°—12° C
Cold	Below 30°C
Mild or cold	30°—33°C
Neutral	34°—36°C
Warm	36°—38°C
Very Warm	38°—40°C
Hot	40°—45°C

Table 15.2 Bath Temperatures

The addition of pine oil, spruce-needles, and chamomile can also aid in relaxation, sleep, healing nervous disorders, skin circulation and the opening of the nasal passages.

The most common types of therapeutic baths are mineral baths with the most common solute being sodium chloride. Other possible cations are potassium and magnesium, and possible anions are chlorine, sulfur oxide, and carbonic acid. Some of these materials will penetrate the skin and will be absorbed by the bloodstream.

Brine baths can be particularly taxing and an hour rest is advisable afterwards.

Athletes should use a warm temperature range mineral bath after training as an excellent warm-down. Sulfur baths are especially help for athletes with joint injuries.

Sports Massage

Sports or athletic massage is performed by a specially trained therapist. This modality is important for stimulating local circulation in especially affected tissues, and to break up muscular knots and metabolic accumulations.

If muscles adversely affected by large training loads are not restored through skillful massage, their ability to contract and function effectively will be greatly compromised. Furthermore, massage, like any other form of restoration, also has an ergonomic effect in that the massaged muscle will expend less energy in the healing process.

One of the advantages of sport massage is that it can deal directly with local areas in need of greater attention than the organism as a whole. Since weightlifting movements have global effects on the body, a severely impacted muscle or muscle group can inhibit the performance of training exercises and hence render the training effect less than optimal. Sport massage can greatly assist in local restoration and consequently allow for global participation.

The field of sport massage is being employed more frequently by professional athletes as competitive levels rise and individuals continue to seek advantages. Sport massage is one of the factors that can affect athletic performance when the training or competitions become especially demanding. It can be a significant factor in allowing athletes to continue preparation at higher levels.

Self Massage

This type of massage can be employed for the restoration of many muscle groups that have not undergone the degree of trauma that results from extreme training. It is economical and convenient and therefore more applicable, especially by athletes who are often traveling or find normal restoration facilities unavailable. This is a form of local restoration that is best applied to those areas that have undergone especially demanding training.

Cryotherapy

Cryotherapy is the process of applying ice to local areas of inflammation in order to minimize swelling through the inhibition of vasodilation. This is especially helpful for local areas that may swell and consequently inhibit the free movement.

The application of ice for 20 minutes, followed by 10 minutes of non-application, is a cycle that can be repeated several times in order to effectively reduce swelling in the aggravated area. For many minor injuries, this simple therapy will allow the body to function effectively at the next training session.

Cryochambers that can maintain very low ambient temperatures have also been found to have beneficial restorative effects on the organism as a whole. More research is currently being conducted in this field and may soon become a significant factor in the entire restoration process. I've recently heard of a cryochamber being manufactured in Germany that can accommodate up to 11 athletes while it drops the temperature 100° below 0 C.

Contrast Showers and Baths

This form of therapy is best performed in a shower room with multiple heads. After a strenuous training session, the athlete showers in water that is set at the highest tolerable temperature possible for several minutes while the adjoining shower is set to the coldest possible temperature. When the athlete's body temperature is well elevated, he or she can then transfer quickly to the cold shower for a period of approximately 30 seconds. This procedure has the effect of first causing significant vasodilation followed by vasoconstriction.

This rapid change does a great deal to enhance the elimination of metabolites from the muscles and thus speed up restoration.

The same durations and temperature ranges can be used for contrast foot baths, which will lead to circulatory improvement in the extremities.

Steam

The use of steam via steam showers effectively raises body temperature and stimulates vasodilation and hence peripheral circulation. The increased body temperature also increases sweating, but the humidity inhibits the loss of heat through evaporation. This causes even more perspiration to take place and thus provides an added avenue of metabolite elimination. Steam rooms and cabinets are not considered effective, as they cannot reach a sufficiently high temperature to penetrate muscle tissue and cause appropriate physiological changes.

Sauna

The dry heat of a sauna is another modality to raise body temperature and increase vasodilation, and thus speed blood flow through freshly trained muscles. The dry heat causes a greater loss of water through evaporation. Again, the influx of blood into the muscles transports in nutrients for the restoration process. A sauna room should be kept between 79° and 96° C. The humidity should range between 5 and 15%.

Apparently, according to my sources, this variation of sauna is practiced in Scandinavian countries. The athletes make use of a sauna that has close access to the outdoors and is put into use during the winter. After a hard workout, athletes disrobe and enter the sauna with the temperature turned up. They then swat themselves and each other with birch twigs for a period of up to 10 minutes. This causes an irritation of the skin that when coupled with the heat of the sauna generates vasodilation to the muscles. After a sufficient heating of the body in this manner, the athletes then depart the sauna and roll naked in the snow.

The sudden cold causes a rapid vasoconstriction that aids greatly in the removal of metabolites from the muscles and hence speeds up the process of restoration. Athletes are much better able to train effectively the following day.

I personally haven't tried this out, but it does seem to be an even more effective means than contrast showers of initiating vasodilation followed by vasoconstriction.

Another effective method is to shower first in 40°C water without wetting the head. Then enter the sauna and sit on the lower shelf for 2 to 3 minutes. After this period, move to the highest shelf and lie down for 6 to 10 minutes. This should then be followed by a 10°C shower of 20 to 40 seconds in duration and then a warm shower of about 38°C for a few minutes. Follow this with a 10 to 15 minute break during which the body is toweled off. This cycle should be repeated for a total of three series.

Swimming

Swimming for short distances in water at a temperature of 27 to 30° C can be especially helpful to relax the muscles after demanding training.

Accupuncture and Accupressure

These two modalities are effective but require professional therapists.

Electrostimulation

Electrostimulation is a particularly effective means of local restoration that is most effective when employed in conjunction with other restoration modalities. EMS units are readily available, but they are only to be used for restoration. Some individuals mistakenly believe that they can stimulate muscular size gains, but this has never been observed in large muscles. Though effective for restoration, they are considered less effective than massage.

Ultrasound

Ultrasound can greatly stimulate local circulation and should be employed to deal with microtraumas. Once instructed properly, athletes can perform their own therapy with this device.

Jacuzzi

The use of hydromassage through Jacuzzi provides a relaxing effect for the muscles while raising the temperature through increased vasodilation. It also provides frictional resistance, which is lacking in other baths. This resistance further increases vasoactivity. This combination of frictional resistance and increased temperature facilitates the influx of nutrients and the elimination of metabolites.

The raising of body temperature and the increase of vasodilation leads to water and electrolyte loss that can have an effect on the metabolic processes that take place during sleep and as precursors to the next day's training. For this reason, water and electrolyte replacement must be considered both in terms of quantities and in timing with relationship to restoration.

Hydration

A person experiences a loss of approximately 2.5 liters of water per day. Some of this occurs during sleep. This loss of water increases the viscosity of the blood. During the course of hard training another 1 to 2 liters of water are lost through perspiration and exhalation. Hydration must be considered as part of the restoration process. The regular sipping of small amounts of water prevents an overfilling of the stomach that may restrict thoracic circulation.

The Future and Facility Design

Anyone planning on designing a weightlifting facility must plan on the inclusion of restoration facilities. Many modern athletic training facilities include an athletic trainers' room that is meant primarily to deal with injuries and rehabilitation. This needs to be expanded to accommodate the aforementioned restoration modalities, and the supervisory personnel must become well versed in their application in order to run a successful program.

The time has passed when a weightlifting facility is just a gym. The facility of the future will be an all-inclusive one suited to effective weightlifting training, general physical preparation, restoration and feeding.

CHAPTER 16
NUTRITIONAL AGENTS AND
THE FEEDING OF THE WEIGHTLIFTER

Although there is no question that a healthful, nutritious diet is of obvious importance to maintain normal health in the organism, it is of even greater value to a hard training weightlifter. There is a high metabolic cost to being a weightlifter, both in terms of caloric expenditure for training, for restoration of the body after training and the maintenance and restoration of the muscles during the periods between trainings.

The topic itself is very complex and in application can be very individualized. For this reason, this chapter will be very generalized and try to touch on concepts that should be kept in mind when focusing on the feeding of weightlifters. This determination of a dietary regimen becomes more specific as the athlete reaches more advanced levels.

At this point, I need to let the reader know that I don't have any special background in nutrition. Most of what I know about the topic is based on my studies of human physiology and the practical experience gained from actually developing athletes. I must include one proviso here for readers who are subject to current popular discussions of the topic of nutrition. Most of the information that is presented in popular media in the United States and countries in danger of being touched by American marketing is geared toward individuals seeking to lose weight and/or body fat. There is hardly ever a discussion available about gaining muscular bodyweight or improving the efficiency of the body in the area of rapid force generation. Consequently, some of the general concepts presented here may seem counterintuitive to readers who are accustomed to conventional wisdom regarding the feeding of human organisms.

The Weightlifting Human As A Digestive Entity

Before embarking further on this topic, it is important to understand the dynamics of the materials that compose the athlete's body. The fairly normal processes of carrying on an active lifestyle requires the constant replacement of materials that are regularly broken down and eliminated by the body's metabolism.

When the task of training the body for competitive weightlifting requires an increase in muscle mass, a strengthening of connective structures, a strengthening and densification of bony material, while simultaneously increasing the metabolic rates of a variety of biochemical processes, it is easier to comprehend the volume of molecular turnover taking place.

All of the metabolic processes, be they anabolic or catabolic, require energy that must come from food sources. So in addition to an increase in the macronutrients, there is also a demand for the micronutrients that facilitate these many metabolic activities.

Fortunately the human species is one of the great omnivores on the planet with a highly adaptable digestive system. The capacity of the body to vary the concentrations and proportions of digestive enzymes secreted is affected by the stressors placed on the body during the training process and thus the chemical digestion and assimilation will be affected.

Because humans walked all over the planet and adapted to a wide range of food-stuffs, they have developed a remarkably adaptable digestive system that can respond to environmental stressors. When humans migrated to a new, previously unoccupied region they probably sampled all the foodstuffs that were accessible. Those that caused a nauseous reaction were probably discarded by the affected individuals, but they remained a possible resource for others. In times of shortage, those individuals with a greater tolerance had an increased chance of survival. Those survivors affected the currently existing human gene pool.

Furthermore, talented weightlifters are exceptionally efficient at digestion and as-similation. For these reasons, an accurate dietary prescription is difficult to develop in light of much of the information regarding diet that is available.

Much of the dietary information that is presently accessible by coaches is not geared toward talented individuals performing prodigious amounts of physical labor at much greater frequencies than has ever been previously imagined. Most "authorities", including some that purport to have expertise in sports nutrition, have had little firsthand experience working with weightlifters competing at top levels. The caloric and protein consumption by competitive weightlifters is significantly greater than that of many other athletes and certainly much greater than the average person.

It is also common to employ some of the strategies that are in vogue with body-builders. Weightlifting and bodybuilding are vastly different in many aspects and as such, their nutritional strategies are bound to differ in very significant ways.

The timing of feeding with respect to training session is another factor that needs to be considered in a chapter on nutrition. The athlete who is training multiple times per day will have specific nutritional needs at different times during the course of the training day. Furthermore, the digestibility and assimilability of the foodstuffs and their timing with respect to training present another factor that must be considered in the strategy. Food that is still undergoing chemical breakdown in the stomach will inhibit or diminish proper training and thus adequate timing must be factored into the daily regimen so that neither training nor feeding must be compromised.

Because of these factors, it is important for athletes to develop daily regimens as they advance through the various sporting classes. As the lifter advances, the number of training sessions, the number and frequency of restoration sessions, and the number of meals increases. Developing a daily regimen that will accommodate all of these demands is absolutely vital for a lifter to continue progress. A haphazard approach will not allow all of the factors to come together and produce a desirable, competitive result.

It is important to realize that a certain number of calories must be ingested prior to the first training session of the day. There must also be time allotted to digestion of breakfast prior to a first morning workout. For this reason athletes must make sure that they sleep a sufficient number of hours prior to waking and eating breakfast. This will allow the daily regimen to begin sufficiently early to accommodate all the commitments of a hard-training weightlifter.

Caloric Intake

A recommended caloric intake for an advanced level weightlifter ranges from 66—77 Calories per kilogram of bodyweight. This is in comparison to a recommended 24 Calories per kilogram of a sedentary individual. These figures may vary as the lifter progresses through a career. Aging, the cycle of training, and increasing bodyweight are all variables that affect the caloric intake. The composition of the diet with respect to macronutrients will also affect the intake of foods.

Macronutrients

Water Water is the most common substance in human protoplasm, composing about 69% of the body. It is dynamic in that it is always leaving the body while more water is simultaneously being absorbed into the body. It performs a wide variety of functions, including serving as a solvent for most solutions, and aiding in thermoregulation and the hydrolysis of large molecules. The body is quite effective at losing and/or eliminating excess water, but cannot compensate well for a lack of water. Of special consideration is the practice of dehydration weight loss in order to qualify for a lower bodyweight class in competition. Although this practice is not frequently undertaken, when it is, the athlete must be rehydrated immediately after the weigh-in in order to avoid cramping and muscle spasms. The procedure of conducting the weigh-in by the time limit one hour prior to the start of competition provides time for feeding and rehydration.

Carbohydrates 10.0— 11.8 grams per kilogram of bodyweight is the recommended range for carbohydrate ingestion. 67% of the carbohydrates should be simple or digestible polysaccharides (starches) in order to meet the energy needs of the athlete. The remaining third should be comprised of dietary fiber for the purpose of aiding in elimination. These fibers actually require energy to move them through the alimentary canal, and subsequently detract from the energy available to the body for training purposes. This elimination is necessary to avoid the putrefaction of fecal matter that could lead to toxicity within the colon and subsequently upset digestion.

The proportion of carbohydrates to proteins should be 4:1 by weight as the simple sugars are the primary source of energy for muscular movements and neural activity. Although both lipids and proteins can be converted to carbohydrates during periods of aerobic recovery, the muscles and nerves require a ready source of carbohydrates in the cells to perform their functions. During protein synthesis, energy largely derived from carbohydrates is necessary to complete the anabolic reactions.

A critical factor to be considered in the feeding of athletes is the absorption rate of materials through the gut wall, and the movement of materials out of the blood stream and into the cells. Easily digested carbohydrates in the form of juices can be administered shortly after training to provide energy for restoration and for the replacement of glycogen (long glucose chains stored in the muscle and liver). The presence of simple sugars in the bloodstream will also stimulate the secretion of insulin, which facilitates the absorption of glucose across the cell membrane.

Fats The normal range of fat consumption for weightlifters ranges from 1.8—2.0 g per kg of bodyweight. Since fats contain 9 kcal per gram compared to the 4 kcal per gram of carbohydrates and proteins, they are especially valuable in fulfilling the caloric needs of the organism during periods of heavy training. Animal fat should comprise 65—80% of the fat intake, and vegetable fats, which contain irreplaceable fatty acids, should comprise from 20—35% of the fat intake. Fats provide essential molecules for hormone synthesis, as well as reserve sources of energy for aerobic respiration during restoration. This is an especially important concept to keep in mind during the training process. The restoration that takes place during sleep and other non-training periods uses energy that is generated aerobically, and fat is aerobically catabolized. Furthermore, fats are necessary for proper brain cell function, and insulation and restoration of the motor neurons.

Because body fat is quite obviously low in some athletes, many aspiring athletes attempt to lower body fat abnormally by limiting caloric intake, especially calories from fats. This is a mistake and can greatly compromise training capacity and restoration. This is part of the syndrome of attempting to replicate the symptom rather than the cause.

Proteins Since proteins comprise 98% of the dry weight of protoplasm, they must be continuously replaced in a healthy, non-training individual. The needs become even more accentuated in hard training weightlifters. The 2.5—2.9 gm/kg of bodyweight required of weightlifters is among the highest ranges recommended for athletes. Not only must athletes rebuild the muscle tissues that are disrupted by training, they must also synthesize the enzymes that keep the metabolic machinery functioning during performance and restoration.

Protein molecules are macromolecules composed of thousands of smaller molecules called amino acids. There are 20 different kinds of amino acids that are involved in the synthesis of proteins. Nine of these amino acids must be ingested: Leucine, Isoleucine, Valine, Lysine, Tryptophan, Threonine, Methionine, Phenylalanine and Histidine. The other eleven amino acids can be synthesized from the essential nine through the process of transamination.

Each protein molecule must be composed of the right number of each kind of amino acids arranged in the proper sequence into order to form the tertiary structure that enables it to fulfill its function as a structural unit or an enzyme. An enzyme is a macromolecule that facilities the assembly or breakdown of other molecules. Since virtually all biochemical reactions in protoplasm are either anabolic (assembly) or catabolic (breakdown), the metabolic machinery is entirely dependent upon having an adequate supply of the proper types of enzymes in the appropriate percentages and at the right time and location.

Ideally the profile of the essential amino acids determines the protein utilization characteristics of the nutrient. The food source having the highest essential amino acid profile and hence the greatest utilization is whey. This means that human tissues are most effectively restored and repaired when the essential amino acids are present in the most ideal ratios, and that ratio is most effectively provided by whey proteins.

Overall, the consumption of a diet that is high in animal-derived proteins and dairy products is an absolute necessity for hard training weightlifters.

Supplementation

Food supplementation is just that—supplementation. It is not meant to substitute for the ingestion of whole foods, but rather as a form of supplying extra amounts of critical macronutrients and micronutrients. Eating a diet composed entirely of whole foods, in spite of the digestive adaptability of humans, is difficult unless the diet is carefully supervised by a dietitian expertly trained in athletic nutrition.

The quality of supplements can also vary by the means in which the primary nutrients are processed, the proportion of the supplement that they comprise, and the other nutrients with which they are combined. Some supplements will also affect how the digestive system regulates the assimilation of certain nutrients and thus, although the quantities of those nutrients may be acceptable or optimal, their assimilation may not be adequate.

Supplements are often easier to digest than whole foods, and as such are more desirable for the hard training athlete that is engaged in multiple sessions per day. For athletes who are training frequently, the amount of time required for digestion and assimilation can interfere with the scheduling of training. Supplements can be processed in order to make these ingestive processes more efficient.

The timing of the emptying of the gut is critical as digestion and assimilation requires a large volume of blood. This blood is necessary for effective training to take place and as such should not be involved in digestive processes, hence the need for supplements that are easily assimilable.

Micronutrients

Micronutrients are vitamins and minerals. Vitamins are organic substances that are required in small quantities to maintain normal health. Minerals are inorganic substances that are necessary in small quantities to maintain normal health. With the development of modern food processing technologies, greater vitamin and mineral supplementation is now an affordable possibility.

While there is a considerable amount of evidence to verify that vitamin and mineral deficiencies may invoke both health and life-threatening consequences, there has not been a great deal of research to determine whether larger dosages are helpful for enhancing the capacity of the organism to withstand greater training stressors.

The timing of dosage with respect to the training and daily regimen is one factor that needs consideration, as is the combination of these supplements with foodstuffs for the improvement of assimilation.

The daily needs of weightlifters for the following vitamins and minerals are as follows according to Volgarev, et al. Many of these dosages can and should be consumed as part of whole foods, but where that is difficult to do or ascertain, supplementation should be considered. Most of these micronutrients are best assimilated when consumed as a part of or with food.

Vitamin C: 175—210 mg
Vitamin B1: 2.5—4.0 mg
Vitamin B2: 4.0—5.5 mg
Vitamin B3: 10 mg

Vitamin B6: 7—10 mg
Vitamin B9: 450—600 mcg
Vitamin B12: .004--.009 mcg
Niacin: 25—45 mg
Vitamin A: 2.8—3.8 mg
Vitamin E: 20—35
Calcium: 2000—2400 mg
Phosphorus: 2500—3000 mg
Iron: 20—35 mg
Magnesium: 500—700 mg
Potassium: 4000—6500 mg

The Daily Regimen

The day's ration of food should be broken up into a breakfast, a second breakfast, a mid-day meal and an evening meal. A snack between the midday meal and the evening meal is acceptable provided that its digestion does not interfere with circulation and respiration during training. The first breakfast should be composed of 20—25% of the day's intake, the second breakfast, 15—20%, the midday meal at 30—35% and 20—25% at the evening meal. Breakfast should be eaten at least 1 ½ hours prior to training, and there should be no more than 12 hours between breakfast and the evening meal. Food should not be consumed too soon prior to training, and not within 20 minutes after training in order to promote sound digestion and to prevent interference with the training physiology.

The various rations of macronutrients should be broken down into proportionate amounts for each meal so that no meal is overloaded in any one macronutrient category. Sufficient time should be scheduled between the last meal and bedtime. Bedtime should be organized so that two hours of sleep are obtained before midnight.

While a lack of proper nutrition may not be immediately or dramatically noticeable, a long-term, improperly-organized diet will interfere severely with the restorative abilities of the athlete's body. This may not impact a single workout, or single day of training, but will over time affect the body's ability to repeatedly meet the demands of heavy training.

SECTION F
CONCLUSION

I commend you, the reader, for having reached this point. You are obviously interested in, and perhaps fascinated by, the process of training weightlifters.

It is my sincerest hope that the information presented in this book will be of great help to you in your development as a coach and that it will be put to good use for the benefit of your athletes. Strange as it may seem, there are people who are merely curious about the process and will read this volume just out of curiosity or because they are simply fans of the sport.

The majority of you, however, are interested in the process, the science and the art of coaching, and you have purchased this book to enhance your knowledge as you undertake the coaching process. Most of you are probably in America or a country with a similar system of athlete development and have limited access to the scant few educational opportunities available for aspiring weightlifting coaches.

Let me begin this section by letting you know that learning about the coaching of weightlifters is an unending, lifelong process and journey. Only a few people have been able to do enough coaching of talented athletes and developed the psyche to generate insightful observations of the process.

There is an academic prerequisite for those truly interested in mastering the art of weightlifting coaching. The aspiring coach must have mastered the reasoning skills of a scientist in order to successfully evaluate new information. Developing these skills is as important a component of science education as is the mastery of the body of knowledge that is relevant to understanding the physical components of the sport.

Part of that scientific education is the time spent with other science students and engaging in stimulating repartee. This is valuable in developing the scientific perspective toward empirical events that take place as a part of the sports experience.

The sports experience is also crucial for a coach since a significant part of the coach's duties is to explain the "feeling" of a particular movement or sequence to younger athletes. Any coach who has not had sufficient experience practicing weightlifting is going to find it difficult to explain feelings. I recall reading a piece on the Soviet method of coaching education. Prospective coaches could only be admitted to the Central Sports Institute after passing rigorous entrance exams in the field of mathematics and science. Those admitted then had to spend the first two years in science courses. At the beginning of the third year they could opt for a particular career pathway, and those that chose to pursue a weightlifting coaching career would then have to demonstrate that they could perform at the Class 2 level. This is not an overly daunting task, but somewhat challenging for those with no special weightlifting talent. This would ensure that they had a familiarity with the training process.

Of course, a considerable amount of effort must be spent in developing appropriate pedagogy and this is best accomplished through mentorships spent with experienced coaches.

Regarding the company of experienced coaches, I recommend it highly. There is no greater way to maintain energy, enthusiasm and the proper mindset for coaching than to engage in conversations with others in the same "profession". Finding out that others are encountering the same problems, or finding out what approaches they've taken to solving them, is empowering. Having your peers recognize your efforts and strategies is equally energizing. These things can only take place through conversations and communication. Even just being a listener at a provocative group conversation can be highly educational and inspirational.

Being a part of the local weightlifting community can also be an educational opportunity. Visiting lifters and coaches from other states and countries may drop by on short notice and might opt for a training session. Only those in the local network ever find out, and often these occasions provide opportunities to mingle and converse with experts. Becoming a weightlifting expert may not be a profession, but it can become an avid hobby that provides an unending stream of learning opportunities.

CHAPTER 17
PATHWAYS

I think that anyone who has gotten this far in this book has a deep interest in pursuing the art and practice of coaching weightlifters. This is an honorable intent if you consider that weightlifting is a sport of considerable value, worthy of being contested in the Olympic Games. In every country outside of America, the national governments have bought into this concept and made it a part of national government policy to keep and preserve weightlifting. At the highest levels, professional weightlifters are coached by professional weightlifting coaches and supported by an infrastructure that seeks out and supports talent.

Chances are very good that anyone young enough to be considering a career and is reading this book will not be able to find a full-time job as a weightlifting coach. There might be a few individuals who will be able to develop a part time weightlifting coaching job, while devoting the rest of their time to running a professional gymnasium that caters to non-weightlifters. In all probability, USA Weightlifting, the national governing body for the sport, will continue to hire at least one-full time professional coach to coach the resident athletes at the Olympic Training Center. In some circumstances, certain individuals have set up full time coaching positions for limited amounts of time. Overall, the employment opportunities do not look especially promising. Most weightlifting coaching in this country will probably continue to be done by well-intentioned amateurs.

Without the prospect of full-time employment, it is doubtful that anyone or any institution is going to be setting up a career education program that might lead to some sort of degree in weightlifting coaching. Why bother? There are several weightlifting coaches in this country who earned legitimate degrees in foreign countries and still can't get a coaching job.

So for those of you who would like to become as good a weightlifting coach as you'd like to be without any prospect of getting a job, this chapter is written with the idea of shortening your educational pathway as much as possible.

Formal Science Education and Formal Coaching

There is no question that you will need to make sure your science education is in place. There's no getting around it. Taking the appropriate college courses is probably the best course of action, even though you think you might have the requisite knowledge without taking the courses.

If you take the courses you will also have to take the laboratory sessions and write up lab reports. This will provide you with the experience of dealing with empirically derived data, and interpreting it. If the course is an excellent one, you will begin to develop some science writing skills that will bring out the objective thinking process. Furthermore, if at some point you decide to apply to graduate school for a Master's or Doctorate in Exercise or Sports Science, you'll find that they're going to require you take these courses at some point along the line—if not before admission, then afterwards.

Courses in biology, chemistry, anatomy, physiology, physics and organic chemistry are the bare minimum. If you are really serious about your preparation, you might want to take further coursework in kinesiology, biomechanics, sports physiology and even statistics.

Now this is beginning to sound like a curriculum for an exercise science major, so you might consider getting an undergraduate degree. At this point you might want to proceed cautiously as the majority of exercise science graduates I've encountered recently have not found their education directed toward competitive athletics. This can find the graduate mentally tweezed off in a pathway that is not especially conducive to developing the instincts of a sports coach.

I would recommend earning a Bachelor's degree in some major, preferably one in the scientific fields, because it will make you more employable in an organization that might be able to sustain your role as a weightlifting coach, even though it may be only on a part time basis. In addition, your degree will qualify you to take the CSCS exam.

There are two good reasons to take and pass the CSCS. It will force you to review the science necessary to pass the exam, and it will qualify you for $3 million in liability insurance. That will cover you in the unlikely scenario that your coaching leads to some sort of liability litigation. Furthermore, it makes you a lot more employable to people that run large organizations. Attending the NSCA events can also put you in touch with some of the top researchers in American Sport Science. They can prove to be valuable resources from time to time.

There are a number of other formal experiences that I would recommend for the upcoming coaches. Attending the three USA Weightlifting coaching clinics, taking the exams and passing them will provide some credibility and lets your prospective lifters and their parents know that you are serious about your passion. It will also put you in touch with other like-minded individuals and the instructor of the course who will, in all probability, be a Class 3 or higher-level coach with a considerable practical background.

A final suggestion is to just talk to coaches from any sport and find out how they are solving the problems of their sport. I've learned quite a bit talking to track coaches, gymnastic coaches, martial arts coaches and others. Some of it wasn't necessarily pedagogy or methodology, but just a different perspective on the development of athletic qualities.

The Avocational Approach

The vast majority of weightlifting coaches in this country have entered the sport through an avocational approach. Some of them might have been physical education teachers or recreational professionals, and chose to coach weightlifting as an auxiliary activity. Others merely fell in love with the sport and put together a gym in the garage or the basement and somehow managed to develop small teams of weightlifters. I was able to start an afterschool program at every school where I worked as a science teacher, and proceeded to develop my skills and weightlifters by putting in lots of volunteer time after school.

Let me warn you that this can get to be a bit of an expensive hobby with the primary benefits being educational and social. Coaching weightlifting can consume big chunks of time, especially if you get involved with hosting competitions in addition to coaching and traveling with your athletes.

If you are strategic about your approach, however, you will develop some great proficiency as an American weightlifting coach, which probably won't be of much value in any other situation. That's OK, though. That can be satisfying enough.

CHAPTER 18
RESOURCES

Within the United States, the available resources for aspiring weightlifting coaches are scant and sometimes difficult to find and subsequently may be difficult to access. In many cases they may not present themselves as directly designated as weightlifting, but in fact may present information that can be used to assist in the development of a weightlifting coach. I'll try to cover the more accessible ones as though I were laying out a course for the most addicted, dedicated prospective weightlifting coach.

USA Weightlifting
http://weightlifting.teamusa.org

USA Weightlifting (USAW) is the National Governing Body (NGB) of the sport of weightlifting, which means it owns the franchise to name the athletes that represent the USA at international events such as the Olympic Games, the International Weightlifting Federation (IWF) World Championships and the Pan American Games and Continental Championships. Through the charter granted by the Amateur Sports Act of 1978, and agreements with the U.S. Olympic Committee (USOC), USAW provides administrative oversight for the sport as they relate to the testing program of the United States Anti-Doping Agency (USADA). It also trains and tests weightlifting officials and subsequently submits the names of those officials for advancement by the IWF. USAW also periodically conducts international competitions, although this is not a direct responsibility.

Although it is not required to do so by charter, USAW conducts a competitive weightlifting program as part of its efforts to produce competitive athletes for international competition. This also allows for the development of coaches and officials. With the exception of national coach Zygmunt Smalcerz, almost all of the athletes, coaches and officials are amateurs.

Although not an educational institution, USAW conducts a coaching certification program that provides education and certification for coaches. It also tests and certifies national level officials. It does not verify empirical knowledge relevant to weightlifting, and subsequently does not disseminate very much training information.

The creation of a Director of Coaching Education position is a move in the direction of sanctioning an approach to the development of weightlifters. As this is being written, a salary has been allocated in the budget for this position. Provided that the position is filled by the right individual, one of the benefits will be that it will recognize authorities in the practice of coaching weightlifters. This will make it easier for aspiring coaches to contact veteran coaches and consult, work with or be mentored by them. Some sort of mentorship program needs to be developed in order for the length of time needed to master the art of coaching is appreciably shortened. This in the long run will shorten the time needed to develop a cadre of elite level weightlifters and hence improve our international fortunes.

A by-product of financing this position is at least a sanctioning of a list of accessible resources that can be relied upon to provide valid information for aspiring coaches. A prominent cause of the current confusion over coaching approaches is the lack of an authority who can certify the reliability of resources.

For the aspiring coach, the competitive program will enable the competitive coaching skills to develop in a formal situation. Furthermore, the competitive events allow members of the community to interact and exchange information, and develop relationships. The best coaches are always present at national events and are usually approachable.

Coaching education seldom takes place in a vacuum, although much of the actual work of coaching takes place in a somewhat isolated fashion. Competitions and clinics allow newer coaches to see the products of experienced coaches and to learn more about the intangible aspects of coaching.

The organization is divided geographically into 43 different local weightlifting committees. Anyone interested in learning more about the sport should contact the LWC chairperson to find out about local events, and then attend them. This will provide an opportunity to get to know people who can be informational resources. It will also enable one to find out about local training facilities and provide an inroad to further knowledge of the sport.

NSCA
www.nsca-lift.org

The National Strength and Conditioning Association (NSCA) is an educational organization that was originally founded to provide some credibility for the Strength and Conditioning profession. It has a strong influence from the sport scientists that have been involved with the organization throughout its early development and in its current manifestation.

The publications regularly generated by the organization, *The Strength and Conditioning Journal* and *The Journal of Strength and Conditioning Research*, contain information that can be very valuable to a weightlifting coach, even though much of it is not especially geared toward the sport. Some of the material is of general value such as the coverage of the effects of certain restoration modalities, or the results of scientific studies that may have an impact on the design of training or coaching.

The NSCA also holds a National Conference, which has a three-day span and features presenters on a wide variety of topics. This can be especially valuable to aspiring weightlifting coaches who are interested in furthering and updating their knowledge of sport science. It also affords an opportunity to meet some top sport scientists and to become acquainted with their programs. More experienced coaches also attend to catch up with professional colleagues and find out about any new research that might have relevance to the sport.

There is a Weightlifting Special Interest Group within the NSCA that can help newcomers with an interest in weightlifting to connect to other members with this common interest. The SIG holds its annual meeting at the National Conference and this opportunity affords members a chance to review the progress of weightlifting as a training modality in strength and conditioning programs.

During the early years of the organization, the influence of a number of sport scientists was instrumental in moving the body away from weight machine training and toward the wider acceptance of free weights and weightlifting movements in particular.

IWF
www.iwf.net

The International Weightlifting Federation, headquartered in Budapest, is the international governing body of the sport. It has a membership of 189 national governing bodies, one of the largest participancies of any sport on the planet. It maintains up-to-date calendars of all international weightlifting competitions and a results section with a great deal of statistical information available for downloads. It also has posted a download of the official rules of the sport.

This is especially valuable for any aspiring coach to maintain familiarity with the top levels of the sport. It is the responsibility of a coach to keep abreast of any rulings or procedural changes that might affect his or her athletes. This includes, but is not limited to, competitive procedural aspects and doping control updates.

For those of you that are fond of keeping track of trends in the sport, the IWF publishes a downloadable result book after every major championship. Since these are all drug tested, the results are as reliable as they can under current standards, and provide an excellent snapshot of the current capacities and trends.

The Internet

Most of you are probably aware that the internet is rampant with would-be authorities, charlatans, and voodoo gurus in just about any field. Weightlifting is no different. There are, however, some legitimate websites that offer quality information and/excellent videos for technical study purposes. I keep an updated list published in my newsletter, and I've reproduced it here to provide a starting point for readers in search of the most recent information.

Helpful Links
One of the suggestions for the Weightlifting SIG was to publish a list of links to websites that contain valuable information for the members. We'll start off with the following. Any others should be submitted to me at info@takanoathletics.com so that I can review them before listing

WONDERLIFTER'S PHOTOSTREAM:
www.flickr.com/photos/wonderlifter/with/7065838187/

PODIUM GOLD WEIGHTLIFTING CLUB ON YOU TUBE:
www.youtube.com/user/podiumgoldwlclub
Interviews with Ivan Abadjiev and videos of some very heavy lifts, the most recent ones of Hysen Pulaku.

DARTFISH VIDEOS OF THE NATIONALS:
http://dartfish.tv/columbusweightlifting
Excellent quality videos of every lift at the 2012 USA Nationals. If you missed the meet, you can see it all here.

TAKANO ATHLETICS:
www.takanoathletics.com
A collection of informative articles and sample training programs, as well as audio interviews with some of the top names in the fields of weightlifting and strength and conditioning.

JOHN GARHAMMER'S PUBLICATIONS:
www.csulb.edu/~atlastwl/JGselectedPubs.html
A compilation of some of John's top research articles. Very valuable stuff.

BRUCE KLEMEN'S FLICKR PAGE:
www.flickr.com/photos/bklemens/collections/
A collection of great weightlifting photos from the top weightlifting photographer in the country.

THE WEIGHTLIFTING COACH ON YOU TUBE:
www.youtube.com/user/robtakano
A brief collection of my lifting videos. Many of these are instructional.

SPORTIVNY PRESS:
www.sportivnypress.com
A collection of articles on Soviet and Chinese training methods as gathered, translated or compiled by Bud Charniga. The Russian Training Manuals and other publications are available for purchase here. Highly recommended by me.

DATABASE WEIGHTLIFTING:
www.iat.uni-leipzig.de/datenbanken/dbgwh/start.php
The statistical results of all major European and international weightlifting competitions since 1973.

WEIGHTLIFTING STORIES AT ESPN:
http://search.espn.go.com/weightlifting/stories/
This page carries some legitimate international and national weightlifting news amidst a good percentage of news stories that use the *weightlifting* tag. Some of the items that fall beneath the radar of many weightlifting aficionados make it on the ESPN page.

1234567898619's CHANNEL at You Tube:
www.youtube.com/user/0123456789619
This channel features Russian telecasts of world championships and other major competitions. Even if you don't understand the Russian commentary, the videos are fabulous, professionally captured and often from several different angles. This is a tremendous resource!

Boffa1226:
www.youtube.com/user/boffa1226
This channel has posted some short videos from the recently concluded World Championships. Excellent footage.

ROB MACKLEM'S Blog:
www.robmacklem.com/blog/
Rob Macklem's excellent photos from the 2011 World Championships. Rob is one of the top lifting photographers in the world.

GUARDIAN:
http://guardian.co.uk/sport/gallery/2011/nov/12/weightlifting
More excellent photos from the 2011 World Championships from a variety of sources including wire services.

OLYMPIC WEIGHTLIFTING.EU:
www.olympicweightlifting.eu
A website with loads of weightlifting videos from high-level competition.

ALL THINGS GYM:
www.allthingsgym.com/2011/11/mens-94-kg-2011-world-weightlifting.html

NEWTON SPORTS:
www.newton-sports.com/public/
Harvey is a long time coaching cohort and his website has a great deal of useful information for those interested in weightlifting or the designing of training programs for strength and conditioning. Harvey is one of the true authorities in our sport. Sign up for the free newsletter!

CATALYST ATHLETICS:
www.catalystathletics.com
Greg Everett's Catalyst Athletics website features plenty of training information for weightlifters and strength and conditioning coaches. Sign up for his free newsletter! Greg also has an excellent e-zine!

DIANNA LINDEN'S SPORTS MASAGE:
www.diannalindensportsmassage.com
Restoration is an absolute necessity for the hard training athlete and no one understands it as Dianna Linden does. Check out this website for helpful information on this much overlooked factor in the development of great athletes.

CRACKYFLIPSIDE'S Channel on You Tube:
www.youtube.com/user/crackyflipside
Over 170 weightlifting videos uploaded, many of them featuring the top lifters in the world. Many of them have bar pathways superimposed providing interesting study materials.

Not everything you'll find on the websites on this list are terrific, but most of it is very helpful and of certain assistance in the education of a weightlifting coach.

CHAPTER 19
CALLS TO ACTION

This book has been written to an audience of weightlifting coaches, potential coaches and individuals who are very interested in the process of training through re-engineering the protoplasm of the organism. For those of you who are truly interested in mastering this process of coaching a weightlifter, there are some driving forces that must be accommodated in order to be successful in this pursuit.

There is no question that there is a huge intellectual component to mastering the art of coaching. A very good weightlifting coach is one who is thrilled with the challenge of appropriately manipulating the various factors that influence performance. Since the sport essentially involves the changing of the physical capabilities of the organism, there must be a tremendous fascination with the normal and extraordinary physiological functions.

Although many of these functions can be studied and learned in an academic setting, the only way to fully understand them is to experience them as they proceed in a talented athlete. In order to understand extraordinary talent, there must be some familiarity with average talent, and as such some coaching work must be performed with those of average talent in order to understand the norms and the extent to which extraordinary talent exceeds those norms.

Competitive Weightlifting as a Participant

This fascination with the coaching process must begin relatively early in life. Hopefully it will be preceded by a passion for weightlifting. Although many exceptional coaches have enjoyed success as an athlete, an equal number of great coaches were far less than stellar athletes. In many cases stellar athletes are so athletically gifted that they have no idea how they achieved their prowess and could not ever explain it or teach it to less talented individuals. Many great coaches are great because they have spent a great deal of time figuring out the best way to achieve improvement and as such have achieved a level of understanding that will be of inestimable value in the coaching process.

The athletic experiences of a coach greatly influence much of the early thinking that provides the foundation for coaching style and approach. For this reason, a coach must participate with great enthusiasm as an athlete during the age range when the best results can be achieved.

Hopefully this participation will take place under the supervision of a knowledgeable coach so that the coaching process can be appropriately modeled. What is important for the prospective coach to internalize from this process of competitive participation, are the feelings that accompany the stresses of training and the return of proficiency during the pre-competition training. Furthermore, the prospective coach needs to experience the anxieties of athletes as they undergo the process of warming up and then learn the art of platform performance. These feelings can only be understood by someone who has undergone the process.

It is only in this way that a coach can internalize the feelings of passion and accomplishment that are essential to the athletic experience. Consequently the coach can develop the psychological triggers that will keep his athletes involved wholeheartedly in the training process.

I feel that participation as a competitive lifter is an absolute pre-requisite for a coach.

Formal Education

Even in a truly amateur coaching situation as it exists in the United States, there is still a need for formal education in certain aspects of math and science. The pursuit of this knowledge need not take place at the very beginning of the pursuit, but it would benefit the coach if some mastery of the subject matter were in place before the study of coaching methodologies begins.

Knowledge of mathematics is not only directly applicable to the task of coaching, but it is also important for interpreting quantitative data that might be presented in regard to training. As an example, a given training variation might produce a different competitive result. A sound working knowledge of the mathematics involved could determine whether the result is significant and whether that variant should be incorporated in future program design. Furthermore, a working coach has to think quantitatively when designing and implementing a training program with a consciousness for the degree of significance each quantity provides.

It should be fairly obvious that some knowledge of physics, biomechanics, anatomy and applied physiology would be of immense value in training program design. After all, a primary actual function of a coach is to re-engineer the protoplasm. The tissues of the body need to be restructured in order to improve their functionality for specific physical tasks. The mechanisms by which this restructuring takes place are well understood by top coaches.

Of course, for these tasks to be carried out, decisions must be made out of an instinctive understanding of the factors. In order to reach this instinctive level of understanding, the concepts must first be mastered, and this can be done most efficiently through a formal education process. University-level courses in these various areas of study would best serve the needs of the aspiring coach.

Just a little side thought that occurred to me after I wrote these last few paragraphs: If you really have aspirations of coaching at the top level, you will be going up against professional coaches from the top weightlifting nations. They are university trained to do what they do. How do you expect to be competitive with these people with an inferior education? Take the courses!

Mentorship

A mentorship is a topic that does not appear regularly in discussions of coaching education, but it is perhaps the one factor that will do the most to shorten the amount of time required to gain the initial levels of coaching proficiency. I was fortunate to have a situation where I was being coached by Bob Hise while I lifted for his team, and I was coaching my own team of junior lifters two or three times per week. Although these two activities took place at different locations, Bob was able to see my lifters competing at local junior meets and then provide me with feedback about my coaching results. This was immensely helpful as it provided me with regular feedback that usually prompted me to alter my strategies.

Because our initial relationship was as coach and athlete, Bob never became hesitant about offering advice, even after I'd reached a certain level of respectability as a coach. This was important, as I've observed many coaches reach a certain degree of proficiency that would in fact isolate them from outsiders who might have valid criticisms of their coaching.

If you, as an aspiring coach, can engage an experienced coach who would be willing to enlist your assistance, the result would be a tremendous boon to your coaching development. Working with new lifters in the development of technique and the remediation of weaknesses while under the supervision of a master coach is precisely the type of supervised training that will lead to a heightened understanding of the process and a mastery of the initial coaching skills.

If the supervising coach can envision the entire training process as a developmental process that will begin with your coaching of the novices, the benefit to your coaching progress will be considerable. Coaching development will take place at a much more rapid rate.

One of the most valuable things that a veteran supervising coach can provide for you is letting you know what to ignore. Two many ambitious novices are anxious to employ and implement every seemingly relevant process to their coaching and no doubt there is an information overload and clutter that makes it difficult to discern a clear pathway. The knowledgeable veteran can be of immense value in prioritizing the efforts of the novitiate, and saving time on the coaching pathway.

Your First Coaching Experience

After you've lifted awhile yourself, worked under the direction of a knowledgeable coach and studied enough of the relevant sciences in order to be literate in technical weightlifting discussion, you should start planning on doing some coaching.

First off, you need to find a facility where you and your prospective athletes will have regular access to the equipment and not feel you are interfering with other activities occurring at the same time. People that want to learn the lifts very badly don't want surprises, so you need to work out the issue of equipment and scheduling as soon as possible. Since everyone's situations can vary greatly, I won't even try to get into specifics.

I would also advise that you consider doing a self-evaluation and find out if your personal characteristics are well-suited to being a coach. One thing that coaches need to possess is better work habits than their athletes. You cannot make demands of people, if you can't initially make them of yourself. Furthermore, you need to set the tone as a role model for your athletes. I've been coaching at a variety of locations and in a variety of situations over my 40+ years as a coach and at no time was I not the individual who spent the most time in the gym. I was there on time for every workout, ready with a training program and ready to get to work. I expected my athletes to be as well.

By the way, when I visited Ivan Abadjiev in Sofia in 1989 when he was coaching the Bulgarian national team, the one thing about which he felt the most pride was that, short of attending major international and national competitions, he had not missed a day in the gym in over 20 years! He was telling me this on a Sunday, and he had given his assistant coaches the day off, while he stayed to watch his athletes train!

Presently there are plenty of people looking to learn how to snatch and clean & jerk that are interested in being coached and don't necessarily know how to verify your credentials, and in many cases don't care. They may be young, old, delusional and in so many ways not ideal, but you should take them on, because they are your learning projects. Of course, don't tell them that, but they are going to present you with a panorama of coaching challenges that you need to learn to face. Nobody with Olympic-type talent and ambitions is going to walk up to an untried novice coach and expect world-class results. You need to start with anyone who will listen to you. But you do need to start.

You probably won't be able to coach more than one or two people effectively at a time. You may think otherwise, especially if you come from a team sport background where technical prowess is not taught very effectively and working in large groups is the norm. The fact is, however, that you, as a novice coach, just don't have the eye to watch a single athlete perform snatches and clean & jerks much less a whole group of people. Start with one or two.

The first big project you've got to undertake (among many small projects) is to teach effective technique. This means that you're going to have to do some diagnosis and begin figuring out where the most emphasis is going to have to lie.

I won't get into technique coaching (because that's a whole other topic for another book), but once you do accomplish that, you're ready to start stealing training programs and trying them out. You need to see how they work, and how you can tweak the programs to make them even better. When you get to that point, you're ready to start using the information in this book and start writing your own.

The Next Step

Of course, you will have to take your athletes to a competition and see how they do. If you are going to be a successful coach, your reputation (and hence your ability to attract more athletes) is based on how well the athletes you coach perform. In order to do that they will have to learn how to perform in a competition, and you will have to learn how to coach them most effectively to do that.

One of the big influences in my lifting career was a fabulous junior lifter from Buffalo named Jack Hill, Jr. Jack was never a full 67.5 kg, but he lifted in that class as an 18-year-old junior and did 117.5 kg and 155 kg for junior world records. Jack in the gym was another story, however. I don't think I ever saw Jack clean & jerk more than 140 kg in the gym. He just couldn't get excited enough in the gym, but on the competition platform he had some big magic. I always wanted to be like Jack, and I think he instilled in me the idea that you should always come up big in a meet. That carried over to how I coach my athletes. To this day, any athlete that trains with me for an extended period of time learns to lift much more in competition than in training, and we are not holding back in training.

If you are going to become a successful weightlifting coach, you must believe that you are largely responsible for the successful result on the competition platform. You will train the athletes, you will help them to develop a regimen that will enable them to train most effectively and you will design the training to ensure that they are physically prepared to peak at the competition. You will also affect their attitudes toward the journey so that they believe that they will be at their best in competition.

After each competition you must determine whether or not your athletes had a successful performance or a dismal one in terms of a number of factors that include personal records, but also technical improvement, performance aplomb and proper attitude. You need to find out what part you played in both the success and shortcomings, and then try to figure how you will change things for the next performance, or if you need to change them at all! Some things you will need to change, and some you will not be able to because they lie within the purview of the lifter.

If you are not one who is given over to self-reflection and self-evaluation, you must develop this mindset, or you will be wasting a great deal of time and effort as a coach. Since you may not have a lot of company as a developing coach, you must find your own way to heighten your abilities to objectively determine the efficacy of your role in the development of your athletes.

Hanging Out With Other Coaches

This is one thing that I believe is a hallmark of other successful coaches and one that is pretty counterintuitive to most of the coaching activities you must master.

Coaching weightlifting is a fairly solitary type of activity and pretty much cloistered. You spend hours and hours in the gym coaching athletes, and very little of what you actually do is made known to outsiders. In the majority of situations you don't have other coaches working with you, and athletes are not your peers. This is important to realize as athletes do and should have other priorities within the weightlifting world. As a coach you are the one largely responsible for the outcomes of your athletes, and you have to deal with those issues on a daily basis. You get used to doing things in a monastic fashion.

For these reasons, hanging out with other coaches is essential for your growth. This generally occurs at competitions, but can take place at organizational meetings, or just through visiting each other's facilities. The important thing is to make these connections and start interacting. Sometimes it is reassuring just to find out that some of the top coaches are having the same problems that you have and they can't figure out what to do about them either.

These interactive sessions are where you are going to encounter concepts, ideas, moods, motivations, attitudes and approaches that are going to shape the way in which you approach your coaching. The actual information about things like technique and percentages is probably not going to be that much of a topic, but rather you will be tapping into a coaching mindset. Once you've made the connection, you will begin to figure out which coaches have the most valuable insights and should therefore be heeded.

Conclusion

When you get right down to it, this is a rather full list of items for someone just embarking on the coaching journey, but all of them are things that will enhance the experience and make it all the more rewarding. This book was written with the thought in mind that the information had not been brought together in a convenient format that could be employed by weightlifting coaches. To use this material effectively you must be a weightlifting coach, and this final chapter was written with the thought of nudging those of you who are not yet coaches to take the first steps. Good luck and I hope you enjoy the journey!

APPENDIX

Sample 20-Week Training Program

This 20-week program was written for my lifters as they trained during the summer of 1998 through the Americans in December of that year. I include this as a study item.

I've also included the spreadsheet analysis that I did in order to keep track of what I was doing. At the completion of this analysis I found that I'd averaged 389 repetitions per week over a 20-week period. For a 50-week year, this came out to 19,455 reps, or a volume that would be appropriate for a Master of Sport class lifter. Most of my more talented athletes made it through this training quite well even though they were doing it under entirely amateur conditions.

What I did was set up a spreadsheet with columns for each of the percentages (intensities). I set up my planned 100% figures for Snatch, Clean & Jerk (cleans and jerks are counted as separate repetitions), Back Squat and Front Squat, and let the spreadsheet do the arithmetic to fill in the figures. Next to each percentage column, I set up columns for repetitions. The spreadsheet also kept track of the repetitions. I had to manually enter the sets. The spreadsheet tallied the total number of sets at the end of each microcycle, mesocycle and the entire macrocycle.

I highlighted the last day of each week (yellow) and the last day of each month (orange) to make it easier to keep track of where I was. The spreadsheet kept track of the totals and averages for each week and month for reps, sets, and load. The last two columns keep track of the average weekly load and the average monthly load. These are calculated by dividing the load by the volume for each time period.

I found that as a result of the final calculation that my K-value was 40.36, which is within the recommended range.

This is a full blown multi-period training program with a down cycle in the 9th week for a meet that was used as a formalized training max-out. The cycle goes back into preparation phase after that brief interlude as squatting returns to the beginning of each workout. The heavier training days in this can be broken up into two sessions per day.

Training Program for the Van Nuys Weightlifting Tribe: 1998 American Open

Week 1
Day 1—Monday, 27 July
1)Back Squat: 60%/4, 70%/4, (75%/4)3   20:20
2)Snatch: 60%/3, 70%/3, (75%/3)3   15:35
3)Clean & Jerk: 60%/3+1, 70%/3+1, (75%/3+1)3   20:55
4)Snatch Deadlift: (85%/4)4   16:71
5)Press: (X/5)4   20:91:91
Abdominals: (X/20)3

Day 2—Tuesday, 28 July
1)Back Squat: 60%/3, 70%/3, (80%/3)2   12:12
2)Power Snatch: 60%/4, 65%/4, (70%/2)3   14:26
3)Power Clean & Jerk: 60%/4+1, 65%/4+1, (70%/2+1)3   19:45
4)Clean Deadlift: (80%/5)4   20:65:166
Abdominals: (X/15)3

Day 3—Wednesday, 29 July
1)Back Squat: 60%/4, 70%/4, (75%/3)3   17:17
2)Snatch: 60%/2, 70%/2, 80%/2, 85%/2   08:25
3)Clean & Jerk: 60%/2+1, 70%/2+1, 80%/2+1, 85%/2+1   12:37
4)Romanian Deadlift (80%/5)4   20:57:213
Abdominals: (X/20)4

Day 4—Thursday, 30 July
1)Front Squat: 60%/4, 70%/4, (75%/4)3   20:20
2)Power Snatch: 60%/4, 65%/4, (70%/3)3   17:37
3)Power Clean & Jerk: 60%/4+1, 65%/4+1, (70%/3+1)3   22:59
4)Overhead Squat: 60%/3, (70%/3)3   12:71
5)Press: (X/5)4   20:91:304

Day 5—Friday, 31 July
1)Back Squat: 60%/3, 70%/3, 80%/3, 85%/1   10:10
2)Hang Snatch: 60%/3, 70%/3, (75%/3)3   15:25
3)Hang Clean: 60%/3, 70%/3, (75%/3)3   15:40
4)Snatch Deadlift on blocks: (85%/4)4   16:56:360
Abdominals (X/20)4

Day 6—Saturday, 1 August
1)Back Squat: 60%/4, 70%/4, 80%/4, 85%/3   15:15
2)Power Snatch.: 60%/3, 65%/3, 70%/3, 60%/3, 65%/3   15:30
3)Power Clean & Jerk: 60%/3+1, 65%/3+1, 70%/3+1,
        60%/3+1, 65%/3+1   20:50
4)Push Press: 60%/4, 65%/4, (70%/2)2   12:62
5)Romanian Deadlift: (80%/5)4   20:82:432
Abdominals: (X/20)3

Week 2

Day 1—Monday, 3 August
1)Back Squat: 60%/4, 70%/4, (80%/4)4   24:24
2)Snatch: 60%/4, 70%/4, (80%/4)3   20:44
3)Clean & Jerk: 60%/4+1, 70%/4+1, (80%/4+1)3   25:69
4)Romanian Deadlift: (85%/5)4   20:89
5)Press: (X/5)4   20:109:109
Abdominals: (X/20)4

Day 2—Tuesday, 4 August
1)Back Squat: 60%/3, 70%/3, (80%/3)2   12:12
2)Power Snatch & Push Press & Overhead Squat:
      60%/3+3+3, 65%/3+3+3, (70%/2+2+2)3   36:48
3)Power Clean & Front Squat & Jerk:
      60%/3+3+3, 65%/3+3+3, (70%/2+2+2)3   36:84
4)Snatch Extension: (85%/4)4   16:100:209
Abdominals: (X/20)3

Day 3—Wednesday, 5 August
1)Front Squat: 60%/4, 70%/4, (80%/4)2   16:16
2)Snatch: 60%/2, 70%/2, (80%/2)3   10:26
3)Clean & Jerk: 60%/2+1, 70%/2+1, (80%/2+1)3   15:41
4)Clean Extension: (85%/4)4   16:57:266
Abdominals: (X/25)3

Day 4—Thursday, 6 August
1)Back Squat.: 60%/4, 70%/4, (80%/4)2   16:16
2)Snatch: 60%/4, 70%/4, (80%/4)3   20:36
3)Clean & Jerk: 60%/4+1, 70%/4+1, (80%/4+1)2   20:56
4)Romanian Deadlift: (85%/5)5   25:81
5)Push Press: 60%/4, 65%/4, (70%/3)2   14:95:361

Day 5—Friday, 7 August
1)Back Squat: 60%/3, 70%/3, (80%/3)3   15:15
2)Power Snatch: 60%/4, 65%/4, (70%/3)3   17:32
3)Power Clean & Jerk: 60%/4+1, 65%/4+1, (70%/3+1)2   18:50
4)Snatch High Pull: (80%/5)4   20:70
5)Good Morning: (X/8)4   32:102:463

Day 6—Saturday, 8 August
1)F. Sq.: 60%/3, 70%/3, 80%/3, 85%/2, 80%/3   14:14
2)Sn.: 60%/2, 70%/2, 80%/2, (85%/2)2   10:24
3)C & J: 60%/2+2, 70%/2+2, (80%/2+2)3   20:44
4)C. H.P.: (85%/3)4   12:56
5)Pr.(X/5)4   20:76:539
Abs: (X/25)4

Week 3

Day 1—Monday, 10 August
1)Back Squat: 60%/4, 70%/4, 80%/4, 85%/4, (80%/4)2   24:24
2)Snatch: 60%/4, 70%/4, 80%/4, 85%/3, 80%/4, 85%/2   21:45
3)Clean & Jerk: 60%/4+1, 70%/4+1, 80%/4+1, 85%/3+1,
       80%/4+1, 85%/2+1   27:72
4)Snatch High Pull: (85%/4)4   16:88
5)Push Press: 60%/4, 65%/4, (70%/4)3   20:108:108
Abdominals: (X/25)4

Day 2—Tuesday, 11 August
1)Back Squat: 60%/3, 70%/3, (80%/3)3   15:15
2)Power Sn. & Push Press & Overhead Squat:
       60%/3+3, 65%/3+3+3, (70%/3+3+3)3   45:60
3)Power Clean & Front Squat & Jerk:
       60%/3+3+3, 65%/3+3+3, (70%/3+3+3)3   45:105
4)Romanian Deadlift: (90%/4)5   20:125
5)Press: (X/5)4   20:145:253

Day 3—Wednesday, 12 August
1)Back Squat: 60%/3, 70%/3, 80%/3, 85%/3, 90%/1   13:13
2)Snatch: 60%/2, 70%/2, 80%/2, 85%/2   08:21
3)Clean & Jerk: 60%/2+1, 70%/2+1, 80%/2+1, 85%/2+1   12:33
4)Clean Deadlift (down in 10 sec): (80%/3)5   15:48:301
Abdominals: (X/25)3

Day 4—Thursday, 13 August
1)Front Squat: 60%/4, 70%/4, 80%/4, 85%/4, (80%/4)2   24:24
2)Power Snatch & Push Press & Overhead Squat:
       60%/3+3+3, 65%/3+3+3, (70%/3+3+3)3   45:69
3)Power Clean & Front Squat & Jerk:
       60%/3+3+3, 65%/3+3+3, (70%/3+3+3)3   45:114
4)Push Press: 60%/4, 65%/4, (70%/4)2   16:130:331
Abdominals: (X/20)4

Day 5—Friday, 14 August
1)Back Squat: 60%/3, 70%/3, 80%/3, 85%/3, 80%/3, 85%/2   17:17
2)Snatch: 60%/3, 70%/3, 80%/3, 85%/3, 80%/3, 85%/2   17:34
3)Clean & Jerk: 60%/3+1, 70%/3+1, 80%/3+1, 85%/3+1, 80%/3+1   20:54
4)Clean High Pull: (85%/4)5   20:74
5)Press: (X/6)4   24:98:429

Day 6—Saturday, 15 August
1)Back Squat: 60%/5, 70%/5, (80%/5)2   20:20
2)Power Snatch: 60%/3, 65%/3, (70%/3)4   18:38
3)Power Clean & Jerk: 60%/3+1, 65%/3+1, (70%/3+1)2   16:54
4)Snatch Extension: (90%/4)4   16:68
5)Clean Extension: (85%/4)4   16:84
6)Good Morning: (X/8)4   32:116:647

Week 4

Day 1—Monday, 17 August
1)Back Squat: 60%/3, 70%/3, 80%/3, (85%/3)2   15
2)Snatch: 60%/3, 70%/3, 80%/3, 85%/2   11:26
3)Clean & Jerk: 60%/3+1, 70%/3+1, 80%/3+1, 85%/2+1   15:41
4)Snatch Extension: (90%/4)4   16:57
5)Press: (X/5)4   20:77:77
Abdominals: (X/25)4

Day 2—Tuesday, 18 August
1)Back Squat: 60%/4, 70%/4, (80%/4)2   16:16
2)Power Snatch: 60%/3, 65%/3, (70%/3)3   15:31
3)Power Clean & Jerk: 60%/3+1, 65%/3+1, (70%/3+1)3   20:51
4)Romanian Deadlift: (85%/5)4   20:71
5)Push Press: 60%/3, (70%/3)3   12:83:160
Abdominals: (X/20)3

Day 3—Wednesday, 19 August
Rest

Day 4—Thursday, 20 August
1)Front Squat.: 60%/4, 70%/4, (80%/4)3   20:20
2)Snatch: 60%/2, 70%/2, 80%/2, (85%/2)2   10:30
3)Clean & Jerk: 60%/2+1, 70%/2+1, 80%/2+1, (85%/2+1)2   15:45
4)Clean Extension: (85%/4)4   16:61
5)Good Morning: (X/8)4   32:93:253

Day 5—Friday, 21 August
Rest

Day 6—Saturday, 22 August
1)Back Squat: 60%/3, 70%/3, 80%/3, 85%/3, 90%/1   13:13
2)Power Snatch: 60%/3, 65%/3, 70%/3, 75%/1   10:23
3)Power Clean & Jerk: 60%/3+1, 65%/3+1, 70%/3+1, 75%/1+1   14:37
4)Romanian Deadlift: (90%/4)4   16:53
5)Press: (X/5)4   20:73:326
Abdominals: (X/25)4

Week 5

Day 1—Monday, 24 August
1)Back Squat: 60%/5, 70%/5, (80%/5)4   30:30
2)Snatch: 60%/4, 70%/4, 80%/4, (85%/4)3   24:54
3)Clean & Jerk: 60%/4+1, 70%/4+1, (80%/4+1)3   25:79
4)Snatch High Pull: (90%/4)4   16:95
5)Press: (X/5)4   20:115:115
Abdominals: (X/25)4

Day 2—Tuesday, 25 August
1)Back Squat: 60%/3, 70%/3, 80%/3, (85%/3)4   21:21
2)Power Snatch & Push Press & Overhead Squat:
60%/3+3+3, 65%/3+3+3, (70%/3+3+3)3   45:66
3)Power Clean & Front Squat & Power Jerk:
      60%/3+3+3, 65%/3+3+3, (70%/3+3+3)3   45:111
4)Clean Extension: (90%/4)4   16:127
5)Good Morning: (X/8)4   32:160:275

Day 3—Wednesday, 26 August
1)Front Squat: 60%/4, 70%/4, (80%/4)3   20:20
2)Snatch: 60%/2, 70%/2, 80%/2, 85%/2   08:28
3)Clean & Jerk: 60%/2+1, 70%/2+1, 80%/2+1, 85%/2+1   12:40
4)Romanian Deadlift: (90%/5)4   20:60:335
Abdominals: (X/20)4

Day 4—Thursday, 27 August
1)Back Squat: 60%/5, 70%/5, 80%/5, 85%/4, 80%/4, 85%/3   26:26
2)Power Snatch & Overhead Squat: 60%/3+3, 65%/3+3, (70%/3+3)3   30:56
3)Power Clean & Power Jerk: 60%/3+3, 65%/3+3, (70%/3+3)3   30:86
4)Snatch Extension: (85%/5)5   25:111
5)Press: (X/5)4   20:131:466

Day 5—Friday, 28 August
1)Back Squat: 60%/3, 70%/3, 80%/3, (85%/3)2   15:15
2)Snatch 60%/4, 70%/4, (805%/4)3   20:35
3)Clean & Jerk: 60%/4+1, 70%/4+1, (80%/4+1)3   25:60
4)Push Press: 60%/4, 65%/4, (70%/4)3   20:80:546
Abdominals: (X/20)4

Day 6—Saturday, 29 August
1)Front Squat: 60%/4, 70%/4, 80%/4, (85%/3)3   21:21
2)Power Snatch: 60%/4, 65%/4, (70%/4)4   24:45
3)Power Clean & Jerk: 60%/4+1, 65%/4+1, (70%/4+1)3   20:65
4)Clean High Pull: (85%/4)5   20:85
5)Good Morning: (X/8)4   32:122:663

Week 6

Day 1--Monday, 31 August
1)Snatch: 60%/4, 70%/4, (80%/4)4   24:24
2)Clean & Jerk: 60%/4+1, 70%/4+1, (80%/4+1)3   25:49
3)Behind the Neck Power Jerk: 60%/3, (70%/3)3   12:61
4)Snatch Extension: (80%/4, 90%/3)4   28:89
5)Clean Deadlift with 2 halts: (85%/3)4   12:101
6)Back Squat: 60%/3, 70%/3, 80%/3, 85%/2   11:112:112
Vertical Jump (X/3)4

Day 2--Tuesday, 1 September
1)Back Squat.: 60%/4, 70%/4, (80%/4)4   24:24
2)Power Snatch & Overhead Squat: 60%4+3, 65%/3+3, (70%/3+3)2   25:49
3)Power Clean & Power Jerk: 60%/3+3, 65%/3+2, (70%/3+2)2   21:70
4)Clean High Pull: 80%/3, 85%/3, (90%/2)4   14:84:196
Abdominals: (X/25)3

Day 3--Wednesday, 2 September
1)Snatch 60%/2, 70%/2, (80%/2)4   12:12
2)Clean & Jerk: 60%/2+2, 70%/2+2, (80%/2+1)3   17:29
3)Power Clean & Push Press: 60%/1+3, 65%/1+3, (70%/1+3)3   20:49
4)Good Morning.:(X/8)4   32:81:277

Day 4--Thursday, 3 September
1)Back Squat: 60%/3, 70%/3, 80%/3, 85%/2, (75%/3)3   20:20
2)Snatch Extension & Snatch: 60%/3+1, 70%/3+1, (80%/3+1)3   20:40
3)Clean & Front Squat & Jerk: 60%/1+3+1, 70%/1+3+1, (75%/1+3+1)3   25:65
Vertical Jump: (X/4)4
4)Snatch Deadlift on block: (90%/4)4   16:81
5)Press: (X/5)4   20:101:378
Abdominals: (X/25)4

Day I5--Friday, 4 September
1)Power Snatch & Push Press: 60%/3+3, 65%/3+3, (70%/2+3)3   22:22
2)Power Clean: 60%/4, 65%/4, (70%/3)3   17:39
3)Clean Extension: (80%/5)5   25:64
4)Front Squat 60%/3, 70%/3, (80%/3)2   12:76:454
Abdominals: (X/20)4

Day 16--Saturday, 5 September
1)Back Squat: 60%/2, 70%/2, 80%/2, 85%/2   08:08
2)Snatch: 60%/2, 70%/2, 80%/2, 85%/2   08:16
3)Clean Extension & Clean: 60%/3+1, 70%/3+1, (75%/3+1)3   20:36
4)Behind the Neck Power Jerk: 60%/4, 65%/4, (70%/3)3   17:51
5)Good Morning: (X/8)4   32:83:537
Abdominals: (X/25)3

Week 7

Day 1—Monday, 7 September
1)Snatch: 60%/2, 70%/2, 80%/2, 85%/2, 90%/1, 80%/2, 85%/2   13:13
2)Clean & Jerk: 60%/2+1, 70%/2+1, 80%/2+1, 85%/2+1,
        90%/1+1, 80%/2+1, 85%/2+1   20:33
3)Snatch Extension: (95%/3)5   15:48
4)Back Squat: 60%/3, 70%/3, 80%/3, (85%/3)3   18:66
5)Press: (X/4)4   16:82:82
Abdominals: (X/25)3

Day 2—Tuesday, 8 September
1)Power Snatch: 60%3, 65%/3, 70%/3, 75%/1, 65%/3, 70%/3   16:16
2)Power Clean & Jerk: 60%/3+1, 65%/3+1, 70%/3+1,
       75%/1+1, 65%/3+1, 70%/3+1   22:38
3)Clean Extension: (90%/3)4   15:53
4)Back Squat: 60%2, 70%/2, 80%/2, 85%/2, 90%/1   09:62:144
Abdominals: (X/20)4

Day 3—Wednesday, 9 September
1)Snatch: 60%/1, 70%/1, 80%/1, 85%/1, 90%/1, (80%/3)3   14:14
2)Clean & Jerk: 60%/1+1, 70%/1+1, 80%/1+1, 85%/1+1,
       90%/1+1, (80%/3+1)3   22:36
3)Romanian Deadlift: (85%/4)4   16:52:196
Abdominals: (X/25)4

Day 4—Thursday, 10 September
Rest

Day 5—Friday, 11 September
1)Power Snatch: 60%/4, 65%/4, (70%/4)3   20:20
2)Power Clean & Jerk: 60%/4+1, 65%/4+1, (70%/4+1)3   25:45
3)Front Squat & Jerk: 70%/2+2, (80%/2+2)4   20:65
4)Front Squat: (85%/3)4   12:77
5)Press: (X/4)4   16:93:299

Day 6—Saturday, 12 September
1)Snatch: 60%/2, 70%/2, 80%/2, (85%/2)3   12:12
2)Clean & Jerk: 60%/2+1, 70%/2+1, 80%/2+1, (85%/2+1)3   18:30
3)Romanian Deadlift: (90%/4)4   16:46
4)Push Press: 60%/4, 65%/4, (70%/4)2   16:62:361
Abdominals: (X/25)4

Week 8

Day 1—Monday, 14 September
1)Snatch: 60%/1, 70%/1, 80%/1, (85%/1, 90%/1, 95%/1)3   12:12
2)Clean & Jerk: 60%/1+1, 70%/1+1, 80%/1+1,
       (85%/1+1, 90%/1+1, 95%/1+1)3   24:36
3)Front Squat: 60%/1, 70%/1, 80%/1, (85%/1, 90%/1, 95%/1)3   12:48
4)Snatch Extension: (95%/3)4   12:60
5)Press: (X/4)4   16:76:76

Day 2—Tuesday, 15 September
1)Snatch: 60%/2, 70%/2, 80%/2, (85%/2)2   10:10
2)Clean & Jerk: 60%/2+1, 70%/2+1, 80%/2+1, 85%/2+1   12:22
3)Clean Extension: (90%/3)4   12:34
4)Back Squat: 60%/3, 70%/3, 80%/3, (85%/3)2   15:49:125
Abdominals: (X/20)4

Day 3—Wednesday, 16 September
1)Power Snatch: 60%/1, (65%/1, 70%/1, 75%/1)3   10:10
2)Power Clean & Jerk: 60%/1+1, (65%/1+1, 70%/1+1, 75%/1+1)3   20:30
3)Push Press: 60%/3, 65%/3, (70%/2)3   12:42
4)Good Morning: (X/4)4   16:48:173

Day 4—Thursday, 17 September
Rest

Day 5—Friday, 18 September
1)Snatch: Same as Monday   12:12
2)Clean & Jerk: Same as Monday   24:36
3)Front Squat: 60%/3, 70%/3, 80%/3, 85%/3, (90%/1)3   15:51
4)Press: (X/3)4   12:63:236

Day 6—Saturday, 19 September
1)Snatch: 60%/2, 70%/2, 80%/2, 85%/2   08:08
2)Clean & Jerk: 60%/2+1, 70%/2+1, 80%/2+1, 85%/2+1   12:20
3)Snatch Extension: (90%/3)4   12:32
4)Clean Extension: (85%/3)3   09:41:277
Abdominals: (X/20)4

Week 9

Day 1—Monday, 21 September
1)Snatch: 60%/1, 70%/1, 80%/1, 85%/1   04:04
2)Clean & Jerk: 60%/1+1, 70%/1+1, 80%/1+1, 85%/1+1   08:12
3)Front Squat: 60%/2, 70%/2, 80%/2, 85%/2   08:20
4)Press: (X/4)4   16:36:36

Day 2—Tuesday, 22 September
1)Power Snatch: 60%/2, (70%/2)3   08:08
2)Power Clean & Jerk: 60%/2+1, (70%/2+1)3   12:20
3)Back Squat: 60%/3, (70%/3)3   12:32:68

Day 3—Wednesday, 23 September
Rest

Day 4—Thursday, 24 September
1)Power Snatch: (60%/2)3   06:06
2)Power Clean & Jerk: (60%/2+1)3   09:15
3)Front Squat: 60%/3, (70%/3)2   09:24:92

Day 5—Friday, 25 September
Rest

Day 6—Saturday, 26 September
Competition

Week 10

Day 1—Monday, 28 September
1)Back Squat: 60%/4, 70%/4, (80%/4)3   20:20
2)Power Snatch: 60%/4, 65%/4, (70%/3)3   17:37
3)Power Clean & Jerk: 60%/4+2, 65%/4+2, (70%/3+2)3   27:64
4)Romanian Deadlift: (80%/5)4   20:84
5)Power Press: 60%/4, 65%/4, (70%/3)3   17:101:101

Day 2—Tuesday, 29 September
1)Back Squat: 60%/3, 70%/3, 80%/3, 85%/2, 90%/1   12:12
2)Snatch: 60%/3, 70%/3, (80%/3)4   18:30
3)Clean & Jerk: 60%/3+1, 70%/3+1, (80%/3+1)3   20:50
4)Snatch Deadlift.: (90%/4)5   20:70
5)Hang Snatch High Pull: (90%/3)4   12:82:183

Day 3—Wednesday, 30 September
1)Front Squat: 60%/4, 70%/4, (80%/4)3   20:20
2)Snatch: 60%/2, 70%/2, (80%/2)2   08:28
3)Clean & Jerk: 60%/2+1, 70%/2+1, (80%/2+1)2   12:40
4)Clean Extension: (85%/3)4   12:52:235

Day 4—Thursday, 1 October
1)Back Squat: 60%/3, 70%/3, 80%/3, (85%/3)4   18:18
2)Power Snatch & Overhead Squat: 60%/3+3, 65%/3+3, (70%/2+3)3   27:45
3)Power Clean & Jerk: 60%/3+2, 65%/3+2, (70%/2+2)3   22:67
4)Romanian Deadlift: (85%/4)4   16:83
5)Press: (X/5)4   20:103:338

Day 5—Friday, 2 October
1)Front Squat: 60%/3, 70%/3, 80%/3, 85%/3, 90%/1, 80%/3, 85%/2   18:18
2)Snatch: 60%/2, 70%/2, 80%/2, (85%/2)2   10:28
3)Clean & Jerk: 60%/2+1, 70%/2+1, 80%/2+1, (85%/2+1)2   15:43
4)Snatch Extension: (90%/3)5   15:58:396

Day 6—Saturday, 3 October
1)Back Squat: 60%/4, 70%/4, (80%/4)2   16:16
2)Power Snatch: 60%/4, 65%/4, (70%/3)3   17:33
3)Power Clean & Jerk: 60%/4+2, 65%/4+2, (70%/3+1)3   24:57
4)Clean High Pull: (80%/4)4   16:73
5)Press; (X/5)4   20:98:494

Week 11

Day 1—Monday, 5 October
1)Back Squat: 60%/5, 70%/5, (80%/5)3   25:25
2)Snatch.: 60%/4, 70%/4, 80%/4, 85%/3, 80%/4   19:44
3)Clean & Jerk: 60%/4+1, 70%/4+1, 80%/4+1, 85%/3+1, 80%/4+1   24:68
4)Snatch High Pull: (85%4)4   16:84
5)Good Morning: (X/6)4   24:108:108

Day 2—Tuesday, 6 October
1)Back Squat: 60%/3, 70%/3, (80%/3)3   15:15
2)Power Snatch & Push Press & Overhead Squat:
    60%/3+3+3, 65%/3+3+3, (70%/2+2+2)3   36:51
3)Power Clean & Front Squat & J.: 60%/3+3+3, 65%/3+3+3,
    (70%/2+2+2)3   36:87
4)Romanian Deadlift: (85%/4)4   16:103
5)Press: (X/5)4   20:123:231

Day 3—Wednesday, 7 October
1)Back Squat: 60%/3, 70%/3, 80%/3, 85%/3   12:12
2)Snatch: 60%/2, 70%/2, 80%/2, 85%/2   08:20
3)Clean & Jerk: 60%/2+1, 70%/2+1, 80%/2+1, 85%/2+1   12:32
4)Snatch Extension: (85%/4, 90%/1)2   10:42:273
Abdominals: (X/25)4

Day 4—Thursday, 8 October
1)Front Squat: 60%/5, 70%/5, (80%/5)3   25:25
2)Snatch: 60%/4, 70%/4, (80%/4)3   20:45
3)Clean & Jerk: 60%/4+1, 70%/4+1, (80%/4+1)3   25:70
4)Romanian Deadlift: (85%/5)4   20:90
5)Press: (X/5)4   20:110:383

Day 5—Friday, 9 October
1)Back Squat: 60%/3, 70%/3, (80%/3)4   18:18
2)Power Snatch: 60%/4, 65%/4, (70%/4)3   20:38
3)Power Clean & Jerk: 60%/4+1, 65%/4+1, (70%/4+1)3   25:63
4)Clean Extension: (85%/4)5   20:83
5)Good Morning: (X/8)4   32:115:498

Day 6—Saturday, 10 October
1)Back Squat: 60%/4, 70%/4, 80%/4, 85%/4   16:16
2)Snatch: 60%/2, 70%/2, 80%/2, 85%/2   08:24
3)Clean & Jerk: 60%/2+1, 70%/2+1, 80%/2+1, 85%/2+1   12:36
4)Push Press: 60%/4, 65%/4, (70%/3)3   17:53
5)Hang Snatch High Pull: (80%/4)4   16:79:577
Abdominals: (X/25)4

Week 12

Day 1—Monday, 12 October
1)Back Squat: 60%/4, 70%/4, 80%/4, (85%/4)4   28:28
2)Snatch: 60%/3, 70%/3, 80%/3, (85%/3)4   21:49
3)Clean & Jerk: 60%/3+1, 70%/3+1, 80%/3+1, (85%/3+1)3   24:73
4)Power Jerk: 60%/4, 65%/4, (70%/4)3   20:93:93

Day 2—Tuesday, 13 October
1)Back Squat: 60%/2, 70%/2, 80%/2, 85%/2, (90%/2)2   12:12
2)Snatch: 60%/2, 70%/2, 80%/2, 85%/2, 90%/1   09:21
3)Clean & Jerk: 60%/2+1, 70%/2+1, 80%/2+1, 85%/2+1, 90%/1+1   14:35
4)Snatch High Pull: (90%/3)5   15:50:143

Day 3—Wednesday, 14 October
Rest

Day 4—Thursday, 15 October
1)Back Squat: 60%/4, 70%/4, (80%/4)2   16:16
2)Power Snatch: 60%/3, 65%/3, (70%/3)3   15:31
3)Power Clean & Jerk: 60%/3+1, 65%/3+1, (70%/3+1)3 20:51
4)Clean Extension: (90%/3)5   15:66
5)Press: (X/5)4   20:86:229

Day 5—Friday, 16 October
1)Front Squat: 60%/4, 70%/4, 80%/4, (85%/4)3   24:24
2)Snatch: 60%/2, 70%/2, 80%/2, (85%/2)4   14:38
3)Clean & Jerk: 60%/2+1, 70%/2+1, 80%/2+1, (85%/2+1)3   18:56
4)Good Morning: (X/6)4   24:80:309

Day 6—Saturday, 17 October
1)Back Squat: 60%/2, 70%/2, (80%/2)3   10:10
2)Snatch Extension: (90%/4)5   20:30
3)Clean Extension: (85%/4)5   20:50
4)Press: (X/4)4   16:66:375

Week 13

Day 1—Monday, 19 October
1)Back Squat.: 60%/4, 70%/4, 80%/4, (85%/4)3   24:24
2)Snatch: 60%/4, 70%/4, 80%/4, (85%/3)3   21:45
3)Clean & Jerk: 60%/4+1, 70%/4+1, 80%/4+1, (85%/3+1)3   27:72
4)Snatch Extension: (90%/4)4   16:88
5)Press: (X/5)4   20:108:108

Day 2—Tuesday, 20 October
1)Back Squat: 60%/3, 70%/3, 80%/3, 85%/3   12:12
2)Power Snatch & Push Press & Overhead Squat:
        60%/3+3+3, 65%/3+3+3, (70%/3+3+3)3   45:57
3)Power Clean & Front Squat & Jerk: 60%/3+3+3, 65%/3+3+3,
        (70%/3+3+3)3   45:102
4)Clean Extension: (85%/4)4   16:118:226

Day 3—Wednesday, 21 October
1)Front Squat: 60%/4, 70%/4, 80%/4, (85%/3)3   21:21
2)Snatch: 60%/2, 70%/2, 80%/2, 85%/2   08:29
3)Clean & Jerk: 60%/2+1, 70%/2+1, 80%/2+1, 85%/2+1   12:41
4)Romanian Deadlift: (90%/5)4   20:61
5)Push Press: 60%/4, 65%/4, (70%/3)3   17:78:304
Abdominals: (X/25)4

Day 4—Thursday, 22 October
1)Back Squat: 60%/4, 70%/4, 80%/4, (85%/3)2   18:18
2)Power Snatch: 60%/4, 65%/4, (70%/4)4   24:42
3)Power Clean & Jerk: 60%/4+1, 65%/4+1, (70%/4+1)4   30:72
4)Snatch High Pull: (90%/3)5   15:87
5)Good Morning: (X/8)4   32:119:423

Day 5—Friday, 23 October
1)Back Squat: 60%/4, 70%/4, 80%/4, 85%/3   15:15
2)Snatch: 60%/3, 70%/3, 80%/3, 85%/3   12:27
3)Clean & Jerk: 60%/3+1, 70%/3+1, 80%/3+1, 85%/3+1   16:43
4)Clean High Pull: (90%/4)4   16:59
5)Press: (X/5)4   20:79:502
Abdominals: (X/25)4

Day 6—Saturday, 24 October
1)Back Squat: 60%/3, 70%/3, (80%/3)3   15:15
2)Power Snatch: 60%/4, 65%/4, 70%/4, 65%/4   16:31
3)Power Clean & Jerk: 60%/4+1, 65%/4+1, 70%/4+1, 65%/4+1   20:51
4)Romanian Deadlift: (90%/5)4   20:71:573

Week 14

Day 1—Monday, 26 October
1)Snatch: 60%/1, 70%/1, 80%/1, 85%/1, 90%/1 (80%/3)3   14:14
2)Clean & Jerl: 60%/1+1, 70%/1+1, 80%/1+1, 85%/1+1,
        90%/1+1, (80%/3+1)3   22:36
3)Snatch Extension: (90%/3)4   12:48
4)Power Jerk: 60%/3, 65%/3, (70%/3)3   15:63
5)Back Squat.: 60%/3, 70%/3, 80%/3, 85%/3, 90%/1, (80%/3)3   22:85:85

Day 2—Tuesday, 27 October
1)Power Snatch: 60%/1, 65%/1, 70%/1, 75%/1, (70%/3)3   13:13
2)Power Clean & Jerk: 60%/1+1, 65%/1+1, 70%/1+1,
      75%/1+1, (70%/3+1)3   20:33
3)Clean Extension: (85%/3)5   15:48
4)Back Squat: 60%/2, 70%/2, 80%/2, 85%/2, 90%/1   09:57:142

Day 3—Wednesday, 28 October
1)Snatch: 60%/2, 70%/2, 80%/2, 85%/2   08:08
2)Clean & Jerk: 60%/2+1, 70%/2+1, 80%/2+1, 85%/2+1   12:20
3)Front Squat: 60%/3, 70%/3, 80%/3, (85%/3)3   18:38:180

Day 4—Thursday, 29 October
1)Snatch: Same as Monday   14:14
2)Clean & Jerk: Same as Monday   22:38
3)Snatch Extension: (90%/3)5   15:53
4)Back Squat: 60%/1, 70%/1, 80%/1, 85%/1, 90%/1, (80%/3)3   14:67
5)Press: (X/5)4   20:87:267

Day 5—Friday, 30 October
1)Snatch: 60%/1, 70%/1, 80%/1, 85%/1, 90%/1   05:05
2)Clean & Jerk: 60%/1+1, 70%/1+1, 80%/1+1, 85%/1+1, 90%/1+1   10:15:282

Day 6—Saturday, 31 October
1)Power Snatch: 60%/3, 65%/3, (70%/3)3   15:15
2)Power Clean & Jerk: 60%/3+1, 65%/3+1, (70%/3 +1)3   20:35
3)Clean Extension: (85%/3, 90%/1)4   16:51
4)Front Squat: 60%/1, 70%/1, 80%/1, 85%/1, (80%/3)3   16:67
5)Good Morning: (X/6)4   24:91:373

Week 15

Day 1—Monday, 2 November
1)Snatch: 60%/1, 70%/1, 80%/1, 85%/1, (90%/1)2, (80%/3)3   15:15
2)Clean & Jerk: 60%/1+1, 70%/1+1, 80%/1+1, 85%/1+1,
      (90%/1+1)2, (80%/3+1)3   24:39
3)Snatch Extension: (95%/3)5   15:54
4)Front Squat: 60%/3, 70%/3, 80%/3, 85%/2, 90%/1, 80%/3, 85%/2   17:71:71
Abdominals: (X/25)4

Day 2—Tuesday, 3 November
1)Power Snatch: 60%/1, 65%/1, 70%/1, (75%/1)2, (70%/3)3   14:14
2)Power Clean & Jerk: 60%/1+1, 65%/1+1, 70%/1+1,
      (75%/1+1)2, (70%/3+1)3   22:36
3)Clean Extension: (90%/3)4   12:48
4)Back Squat: 60%/2, 70%/2, 80%/2, 85%/2, 90%/2   10:58:129
Abdominals: (X/20)4

Day 3—Wednesday, 4 November
1)Snatch: 60%/1, 70%/1, 80%/1, 85%/1, 90%/1   05:05
2)Clean & Jerk: 60%/1+1, 70%/1+1, 80%/1+1, 85%/1+1, 90%/1+1   10:15
3)Snatch Extension: (90%/3)4   12:27
4)Front Squat: 60%/2, 70%/2, 80%/2, 85%/2, 90%/2   10:37:166
Abdominals: (X/25)4

Day 4—Thursday, 5 November
1)Power Snatch: 60%/2, 65%/2, (70%/2)2   08:08
2)Power Clean & Jerk: 60%/2+1, 65%/2+1, (70%/2+1)2   12:20
3)Clean Extension: (85%/3)4   12:32:198
Abdominals: (X/25)4

Day 5—Friday, 6 November
Rest

Day 6—Saturday, 7 November
Competition

Week 16

Day 1—Monday, 9 November
1)Snatch: 60%/1, 70%/1, 80%/1, 85%/1, (90%/1)3, (80%/3)3   16:16
2)Clean & Jerk: 60%/1+1, 70%/1+1, 80%/1+1, 85%/1+1,
        (90%/1+1)3, (80%/3+1)3   26:42
3)Snatch Extension: (100%/3)4   12:54
4)Front Squat.: 60%/1, 70%/1, 80%/1, 85%/1, (90%/1)3, (80%/3)3   16:70
5)Press: (X/4)4   16:86:86

Day 2—Tuesday, 10 November
1)Snatch: 60%/2, 70%/2, (80%/2)4   12:12
2)Clean & Jerk: 60%/2+1, 70%/2+1, (80%/2+1)4   18:30
3)Clean Extension: (90%/3)4   12:42
4)Front Squat: 60%/3, 70%/3, (80%/3)3   15:57:143
Abdominals: (X/20)4

Day 3—Wednesday, 11 November
1)Power Snatch: 60%/1, 65%/1, 70%/1, 75%/1, (70%/3)3   13:13
2)Power Clean & Jerk: 60%/1+1, 65%/1+1, 70%/1+1,
        75%/1+1, (70%/3+1)3   20:33
3)Back Squat: 60%/3, 70%/3, 80%/3, 85%/3, 90%/1   13:46:189
Abdominals: (X/25)4

Day 4—Thursday, 12 November
Rest

Day 5—Friday, 13 November
1)Snatch: 60%/1, 70%/1, 80%/1, 85%/1, 90%/1, 80%/1, 85%/1   07:07
2)Clean & Jerk: 60%/1+1, 70%/1+1, 80%/1+1, 85%/1+1,
       90%/1+1, 80%/1+1, 85%/1+1   14:21
3)Snatch Extension: (100%/3)5   15:36
4)Front Squat: 60%/2, 70%/2, 80%/2, 85%/2, 90%/2, 80%/2, 85%/2   14:50
5)Press: (X/5)4   20:70:259
Abdominals: (X/25)4

Day 6—Saturday, 14 November
1)Power Snatch: 60%/2, 65%/2, 70%/2, 65%/2, 70%/2   10:10
2)Power Clean & Jerk: 60%/2+1, 65%/2+1, 70%/2+1,
       65%/2+1, 70%/2+1   15:25
3)Clean Extension: (90%/3)4   12:37
4)Back Squat: 60%/3, 70%/3, 80%/3, (85%/3, 90%/1, 95%/1)3   24:61
5)Good Morning: (X/5)4   20:81:340

Week 17

Day 1—Monday, 16 November
1)Snatch: 60%/1, 70%/1, 80%/1, (85%/1, 90%/1, 95%/1)3   12:12
2)Clean & Jerk: 60%/1+1, 70%/1+1, 80%/1+1,
       (85%/1+1, 90%/1+1, 95%/1+1)3   24:36
3)Snatch Extension: (95%/3)5   15:51
4)Front Squat: Same as Snatch   12:63
5)Press: (X/3)4   12:75:75

Day 2—Tuesday, 17 November
1)Snatch: 60%/2, 70%/2, 80%/2, 85%/2   08:08
2)Clean & Jerk: 60%/2+1, 70%/2+1, 80%/2+1, 85%/2+1   12:20
3)Clean Extension: (90%/3)5   15:35
4)Front Squat: 60%/2, 70%/2, 80%/2, 85%/2, 80%/2   10:45:120
Abdominals: (X/20)4

Day 3—Wednesday, 18 November
1)Power Snatch: 60%/1, (65%/1, 70%/1, 75%/1)3   10:10
2)Power Clean & Jerk: 60%/1+1, (65%/1+1, 70%/1+1, 75%/1+1)3   20:30
3)Power Jerk: 60%/3, 65%/3, (70%/3)3   15:45
4)Back Squat: 60%/2, 70%/2, 80%/2, 85%/2, 90%/1   09:54:174

Day 4—Thursday, 19 November
Rest

Day 5—Friday, 20 November
1)Snatch: Same as Monday   12:12
2)Clean & Jerk: Same as Monday   24:36
3)Snatch High Pull: (90%/3)5   15:51
4)Front Squat: 60%/2, 70%/2, 80%/2, 85%/2, 90%/2, 95%/1   11:62
5)Good Morning: (X/4)4 16:78:252

Day 6—Saturday, 21 November
1)Power Snatch: 60%/2, 65%/2, (70%/2)3   10:10
2)Power Clean & Jerk: 60%/2+1, 65%/2+1, (70%/2+1)3   15:25
3)Front Squat & Jerk: (80%/2+2)4   16:41
4)Back Squat: 60%/3, 70%/3, 80%/3, 85%/3, 90%/2, 80%/3, 85%/2   19:60
5)Press: (X/4)4   16:76:328
Abdominals: (X/25)4

Week 18

Day 1—Monday 23 November
1)Snatch Singles to max (max-10, max-5, max)2   12:12
2)Clean & Jerk: Singles to max (max-10, max-5, max)2   24:36
3)Snatch Extension: (100%/2)4   08:44
4)Front Squat: Singles to max, (max-10, max-5, max)2   12:56:56

Day 2—Tuesday, 24 November
1)Snatch: 60%/2, 70%/2, 80%/2, (85%/2)2   10:10
2)Clean & Jerk: 60%/2+1, 70%/2+1, 80%/2+1, (85%/2+1)2   15:25
3)Clean Extension: (95%/2)4   08:33
4)Good Morning: (X/4)4   16:49:105

Day 3—Wednesday, 25 November
1)Power Snatch: Singles to max, (max-10, max-5, max)2   11:11
2)Power Clean & Jerk: Singles to max, (max-10, max-5, max)   22:33
3)Back Squat: 60%/2, 70%/2, 80%/2, 85%/2, 90%/2, 95%/1   11:44
4)Press: (X/3)4   12:56:161

Day 4—Thursday, 26 November
Rest

Day 5—Friday, 27 November
1)Snatch: Same as Monday   12:12
2)Clean & Jerk:Same as Monday   24:36
3)Front Squat: Same as Monday   12:48
4)Snatch Extension: (100%/2)4   08:56:217

Day 6—Saturday, 28 November
1)Power Snatch: Same as Wednesday   11:11
2)Power Clean & Jerk: Same as Wednesday   22:33
3)Press: (X/3)4   12:45:262

Week 19

Day 1—Monday, 30 November
1)Snatch: Singles to max, (max-10, max-5, max)   9:9
2)Clean & Jerk: Singles to max, (max-10, max-5, max)   18:27
3)Front Squat: Singles to max (max-10, max-5, max)   9:36:36

Day 2—Tuesday, 1 December
1)Power Snatch: 60%/2, (65%/2, 70%/2, 75%/1)3   17:17
2)Power Clean & Jerk: 60%/2+1, (65%/2+1, 70%/2+1, 75%/1+1)3   27:44
3)Back Squat: 60%/3, 70%/3, 80%/3, (85%/3)3   18:62:98

Day 3—Wednesday, 2 December
Rest

Day 4—Thursday, 3 December
1)Snatch: 60%/1, 70%/1, 80%/1, 85%/1, 90%/1, 85%/1   06:06
2)Clean & Jerk: 60%/1+1, 70%/1+1, 80%/1+1, 85%/1+1,
          90%/1+1, 85%/1+1   12:28
3)Snatch Extension: (100%/2)4   08:36
4)Front Squat: 60%/2, 70%/2, 80%/2, 85%/2, (90%/2)2   12:48:146

Day 5—Friday, 4 December
Rest

Day 6—Saturday, 5 December
1)Snatch: 60%/2, 70%/2, 80%/2, 85%/2   08:08
2)Clean & Jerk: 60%/2+1, 70%/.2+1, 80%/2+1, 85%/2+1   12:20
3)Clean Extension: (85%/3)4   12:32
4)Press: (X/3)4   12:44:190

Week 20

Day 1—Monday, 7 December
1)Snatch: 60%/1, 70%/1, 80%/1, 85%/1   04:04
2)Clean & Jerk: 60%/1+1, 70%/1+1, 80%/1+1, 85%/1+1   08:12
3)Front Squat: 60%/2, 70%/2, 80%/2, 85%/2   08:20
4)Press: (X/3)4   12:32:32

Day 2—Tuesday, 8 December
1)Power Snatch: 60%/2, 65%/2, 70%/1   05:05
2)Power Clean & Jerk: 60%/2+1, 65%/2+1, 70%/1+1   08:13:45

Day 3—Wednesday, 9 December
1)Power Snatch: (60%/2)3   06:06
2)Power Clean & Jerk: (60%/2+1)3   09:15
3)Jumping Back Squat: (50%/2)3   06:21:66

Day 4—Thursday, 10 December
Rest

Day 5—Friday, 11 December
Activity?

Day 6 or 7
Competition

Table A.1 20-Week Program Excel Analysis: Week 1

Wk	Day	Order	Exercise	60%	R	65%	R	70%	R	75%	R	80%	R	85%	R	90%	R	95%	R	100%	R	105%	R	Vol	Dvol	Wvol	Mvol	Load	Dload	WkLoad	MoLoad	Sets	Dsets	WkSets	MoSets	WkAvl	MAvl
1	1	1	Back Squat	150	4	163		175	4	188	12	200		213		225		238		250		263		20				3550				5					
1	1	2	Snatch	78	3	85		91	3	98	9	104		111		117		124		130		137		15				1364.5				5					
1	1	3a	Clean	96	3	104		112	3	120	9	128		136		144		152		160		168		15				1704				5					
1	1	3b	Jerk	96	1	104		112	1	120	3	128		136		144		152		160		168		5				568									
1	1	4	Snatch Deadlift	78		85		91		98		104	16	111		117		124		130		137		16				1768				4					
1	1	5	Press	54		59		63		68		72	20	77		81		86		90		95		20	91			1350	10325			4	23				
1	2	1	Back Squat	150	3	163		175	3	188		200	6	213		225		238		250		263		12				2175				4					
1	2	2	Power Snatch	78	4	85		91	4	98		104		111		117		124		130		137		14				1196				5					
1	2	3a	Power Clean	96	4	104		112	4	120		128		136		144		152		160		168		14				1472				5					
1	2	3b	Jerk	96	1	104		112	1	120	3	128		136		144		152		160		168		5				536									
1	2	4	Clean Deadlift	96		104		112		120		128	20	136	20	144		152		160		168		20	65			2560	7939			4	18				
1	3	1	Back Squat	150		163		175		188		200		213		225		238		250		263		21				4200				5					
1	3	2	Snatch	78	2	85		91	2	98		104		111		117		124		130		137		8				767				4					
1	3	3a	Clean	96	2	104		112	2	120		128		136		144		152		160		168		8				944				4					
1	3	3b	Jerk	96	1	104		112	1	120		128		136		144		152		160		168		4				472									
1	3	4	Romanian Deadlift	96		104		112		120		128	20	136	20	144		152		160		168		20	61			2560	8943			4	17				
1	4	1	Front Squat	120	4	130		140	4	150	12	160		170		180		190		200		210		20				2840				5					
1	4	2	Power Snatch	78		85		91		98		104		111		117		124		130		137		17				1469				5					
1	4	3a	Power clean	96		104		112		120		128		136		144		152		160		168		17				1808				5					
1	4	3b	Jerk	96	1	104		112	1	120	3	128		136		144		152		160		168		5				536									
1	4	4	Overhead Squat	78	3	85		91	3	98		104		111		117		124		130		137		12				1053				4					
1	4	5	Press	54		59		63		68		72	20	77		81		86		90		95		20	91			1350	9056			4	23				
1	5	1	Back Squat	150	3	163		175	3	188		200		213		225		238		250		263		10				1787.5				4					
1	5	2	Hang Snatch	78	3	85		91	3	98	9	104		111		117		124		130		137		15				1384.5				5					
1	5	3a	Hang Clean	96	3	104		112	3	120	9	128		136		144		152		160		168		15				1704				5					
1	5	4	Snatch Deadlift on blocks	78		85		91		98		104	16	111		117		124		130		137		16	56			1768	6644			4	18				
1	6	1	Back Squat	150	4	163		175	4	188		200		213		225		238		250		263		15				2737.5				4					
1	6	2	Power Snatch	78	6	85		91		98		104		111		117		124		130		137		15				1248				5					
1	6	3a	Power Clean	96	6	104		112	6	120		128		136		144		152		160		168		15				1536				5					
1	6	3b	Jerk	96	1	104		112	2	120		128		136		144		152		160		168		5				512									
1	6	4	Push Press	78	4	85		91	4	98		104		111		117		124		130		137		12				1248				4					
1	6	5	Romanian Deadlift	96	4	104		112	4	120		128	20	136	20	144		152		160		168		20	82	446		2560	9842	43773.5		4	22	102		98.1	

Table A.1 20-Week Program Excel Analysis: Week 2

Wk	Day	Order	Exercise	60%	R	65%	R	70%	R	75%	R	80%	R	85%	R	90%	R	95%	R	100%	R	105%	R	Vol	Dvol	Wvol	Mvol	Load	Dload	WkLoad	MoLoad	Sets	Dsets	WkSets	MoSets	WkAvl	MAvl
2	1	1	Back Squat	150	4	163		175		188	4	200	16	213		225		238		250		263		24				4500				6					
2	1	2	Clean	78		85		91		98		104		111		117		124		130		137		20				1924				5					
2	1	3a	Clean	96		104		112		120		128		136		144		152		160		168		20				2368				5					
2	1	3b	Jerk	96		104		112		120		128		136		144		152		160		168		5				592									
2	1	4	Romanian Deadlift	96		104		112		120		128	20	136		144		152		160		168		20				2720				4					
2	1	5	Press	54		59		63		68	20	72		77		81		86		90		95		20	109			1350	13454			4	24				
2	2	1	Back Squat	150		163		175		188		200		213		225		238		250		263		12				2175				4					
2	2	2a	Power Snatch	78		85		91		98		104		111		117		124		130		137		12				1033.5				5					
2	2	2b	Behind Neck Push Press	78		85		91		98		104		111		117		124		130		137		12				1033.5									
2	2	2c	Overhead Squat	78		85		91		98		104		111		117		124		130		137		12				1033.5									
2	2	3a	Power Clean	96		104		112		120		128		136		144		152		160		168		12				1272				5					
2	2	3b	Front Squat	96		104		112		120		128		136		144		152		160		168		12				1272									
2	2	3c	Jerk	96		104		112		120		128		136		144		152		160		168		12				1272									
2	2	4	Snatch Extension	78		85		91		98		104		111	16	117		124		130		137		16	100			1768	10860			4	18				
2	3	1	Front Squat	120		130		140		150		160		170		180		190		200		210		16				2320				4					
2	3	2	Snatch	78		85		91		98		104		111		117		124		130		137		20				1924				5					
2	3	3a	Clean	96		104		112		120		128		136		144		152		160		168		16				1856				4					
2	3	3b	Jerk	96		104		112		120		128		136		144		152		160		168		4				464									
2	3	4	Clean Extension	96		104		112		120		128		136	16	144		152		160		168		16	72			2176	8740			4	17				
2	4	1	Back Squat	150		163		175		188		200		213		225		238		250		263		16				2900				4					
2	4	2	Snatch	78		85		91		98		104		111		117		124		130		137		20				1924				5					
2	4	3a	Clean	96		104		112		120		128		136		144		152		160		168		16				1856				4					
2	4	3b	Jerk	96		104		112		120		128		136		144		152		160		168		4				464									
2	4	4	Romanian Deadlift	96		104		112		120		128	25	136		144		152		160		168		25				3400				5					
2	4	5	Push Press	96		104		112		120		128		136		144		152		160		168		14	95			1472	12016			4	22				
2	5	1	Back Squat	150		163		175		188		200		213		225		238		250		263		15				2775				5					
2	5	2	Power Snatch	78		85		91		98		104		111		117		124		130		137		17				1469				5					
2	5	3a	Power Clean	96		104		112		120		128		136		144		152		160		168		14				1472				4					
2	5	3b	Jerk	96		104		112		120		128		136		144		152		160		168		4				424									
2	5	4	Snatch High Pull	78		85		91		98		104	20	111		117		124		130		137		20				2080				4					
2	5	5	Good morning	48		52		56		60		64		68		72		76		80	32	84		32	102			2560	10780			4	22				
2	6	1	Front Squat	120		130		140		150		160		170		180		190		200		210		14				2080				5					
2	6	2	Snatch	78		85		91		98		104		111		117		124		130		137		10				988				5					
2	6	3a	Clean	96		104		112		120		128		136		144		152		160		168		10				1184				5					
2	6	3b	Jerk	96		104		112		120		128		136		144		152		160		168		10				1184									
2	6	4	Clean High Pull	96		104		112		120		128		136		144	12	152		160		168		12				1632				4					
2	6	5	Press	54		59		63		68		72		77		81		86		90		95		20	76	554		1350	8418	64267.5		4	23	126			110.8

Table A.1 20-Week Program Excel Analysis: Week 3

Wk	Day	Order	Exercise	60%	R	65%	70%	R	75%	R	80%	R	85%	R	90%	R	95%	R	100%	R	105%	R	Vol	Dvol	Wvol	Load	Dload	WkLoad	Sets	Dsets	WkSets	MAvl
3	1	1	Back Squat	150	4	163	175	4	188	4	200	12	213		225	4	238		250		263		24			4550			6			
3	1	2	Snatch	78	4	85	91	4	98		104	8	111	5	117	5	124		130		137		21			2060.5			6			
3	1	3a	Clean	96	4	104	112	4	120		128	8	136	8	144	2	152		160		168		21			2536			6			
3	1	3b	Jerk	96		104	112	1	120	1	128	2	136		144	1	152		160		168		6			736						
3	1	4	Snatch High Pull	78		85	91		98		104		111		117	16	124		130		137		16			1768			4			
3	1	5	Push Press	96	4	104	112	12	120		128		136		144		152		160		168		20	108		2144	13795		5	27		
3	2	1	Back Squat	150	3	163	175	3	188		200	9	213		225		238		250		263		15			2775			5			
3	2	2a	Power Snatch	78	3	85	91	3	98		104	2	111		117		124		130		137		15			1306.5			5			
3	2	2b	Behind Neck Push Press	78	3	85	91	3	98		104	2	111		117		124		130		137		15			1306.5						
3	2	2c	Overhead Squat	78	3	85	91	3	98		104	2	111		117		124		130		137		15			1306.5						
3	2	3a	Power Clean	96	3	104	112	3	120		128	3	136		144		152		160		168		15			1608			5			
3	2	3b	Front Squat	96	3	104	112	3	120		128	3	136		144		152		160		168		15			1608						
3	2	3c	Jerk	96	3	104	112	3	120		128	3	136		144		152		160		168		15			1608						
3	2	4	Romanian Deadlift	96		104	112		120		128		136		144	20	152		160		168		20			2880			5			
3	2	5	Press	54		59	63		68		72	20	77		81		86		90		95		20	145		1440	15839		4	24		
3	3	1	Back Squat	150	3	163	175	3	188		200	3	213		225	1	238		250		263		13			2437.5			5			
3	3	2	Snatch	78	3	85	91	2	98		104	2	111		117		124		130		137		8			767			4			
3	3	3a	Clean	96	3	104	112	2	120		128	2	136		144		152		160		168		8			944			4			
3	3	3b	Jerk	96		104	112	1	120		128	1	136		144	1	152		160		168		4			472						
3	3	4	Eccentric Clean Deadlift	96		104	112		120		128	15	136		144		152		160		168		15	48		1920	6541		5	18		
3	4	1	Front Squat	120	4	130	140	4	150		160	12	170		180	4	190		200		210		24			3640			6			
3	4	2a	Power Snatch	78	3	85	91	3	98		104	2	111		117		124		130		137		15			1306.5			5			
3	4	2b	Behind Neck Push Press	78	3	85	91	3	98		104	2	111		117		124		130		137		15			1306.5						
3	4	2c	Overhead Squat	78	3	85	91	3	98		104	2	111		117		124		130		137		15			1306.5						
3	4	3a	Power Clean	96	3	104	112	3	120		128	3	136		144		152		160		168		15			1608			5			
3	4	3b	Front Squat	96	3	104	112	3	120		128	3	136		144		152		160		168		15			1608						
3	4	3c	Jerk	96	3	104	112	3	120		128	3	136		144		152		160		168		15			1608						
3	4	4	Push Press	96	4	104	112	8	120		128		136		144		152		160		168		16	130		1696	14090		4	20		
3	5	1	Back Squat	150	5	163	175	5	188		200	6	213		225		238		250		263		17			3237.5			6			
3	5	2	Snatch	78	3	85	91	12	98		104	6	111		117		124		130		137		17			1683.5			6			
3	5	3a	Clean	96	3	104	112	6	120		128	6	136		144		152		160		168		15			1800			5			
3	5	3b	Jerk	96		104	112	2	120		128	2	136		144	1	152		160		168		5			600						
3	5	4	Clean High Pull	78		85	91		98		104		111		117	16	124	16	130		137		20			2720			5			
3	5	5	Press	54		59	63		68		72	20	77		81		86		90		95		20	94		1440	11481		4	26		
3	6	1	Back Squat	150	5	163	175		188		200	10	213		225		238		250		263		20			3625			4			
3	6	2	Power Snatch	78	3	85	91	12	98		104	6	111		117		124		130		137		18			1579.5			6			
3	6	3a	Power Clean	96	3	104	112	6	120		128	6	136		144		152		160		168		12			1272			4			
3	6	3b	Jerk	96		104	112	2	120	2	128		136		144		152		160		168		4			424						
3	6	4	Snatch Extension	78		85	91		98		104		111		117	16	124	16	130		137		16			1872			4			
3	6	5	Clean Extension	96		104	112		120		128		136		144		152		160		168		16			2176			4			
3	6	6	Good Morning	48		52	56		60		64		68		72	16	76		80		84		32	118	643	2560	13509	75242.5	4	26	141	117.0

Table A.1 20-Week Program Excel Analysis: Week 4

Wk	Day	Order	Exercise	60%	R	65%	R	70%	R	75%	R	80%	R	85%	R	90%	R	95%	R	100%	R	105%	R	Vol	Dvol	Vvol	Mvol	Load	Dload	WtLoad	MoLoad	Sets	Dsets	WkSets	MoSets	WkAvl	MAvl
4	1	1	Back Squat	150	3	163		175		188	3	200	3	213	3	225	6	238		250		263		15				2850				5					
4	1	2	Snatch	78	3	85		91	3	98	3	104	3	111	3	117	2	124		130		137		11				1040				4					
4	1	3a	Clean	96		104		112		120	3	128	3	136	3	144	2	152		160		168		11				1280				4					
4	1	3b	Jerk	78		85		91		98	1	104	1	111	1	117	1	124		130		137		4				472									
4	1	4	Snatch Extension															124	16	130		137		16				1872				4					
4	1	5	Press	54		59		63		68		72	20	77		81		86		90		95		20	77			1440	8954			4	21				
4	2	1	Back Squat	150	4	163		175		188	4	200	8	213		225		238		250		263		16				2900				4					
4	2	2	Power Snatch	78	3	85	3	91		98	9	104		111		117		124		130		137		15				1306.5				5					
4	2	3a	Power Clean	96	3	104	3	112	3	120	9	128		136		144		152		160		168		15				1608				5					
4	2	3b	Jerk	96	1	104	1	112	1	120	3	128		136		144		152		160		168		5				536									
4	2	4	Romanian Deadlift	96		104		112		120		128	20	136		144	20	152		160		168		20				2720				4					
4	2	5	Push Press	96	3	104	3	112	9	120		128		136		144		152		160		168		12	83			1296	10367			4	22				
4	4	1	Front Squat	120	4	130	2	140	4	150	4	160	12	170	2	180		190		200		210		20				2960				5					
4	4	2	Snatch	78	2	85	2	91	2	98	2	104	2	111	2	117	4	124		130		137		10				988				5					
4	4	3a	Clean	96	2	104	2	112	2	120	2	128	2	136	2	144	4	152		160		168		10				1216				5					
4	4	3b	Jerk	96	1	104	1	112	1	120	1	128	3	136		144		152		160		168		5				592									
4	4	4	Clean Extension	96		104		112		120		128		136	16	144	16	152		160		168		16				2176				4					
4	4	5	Good Morning	48		52		56		60		64		68		72		76		80	32	84		32	93			2560	10492			4	23				
4	6	1	Back Squat	150	3	163	3	175		188	3	200	3	213	3	225	3	238	1	250		263		13				2437.5				5					
4	6	2	Power Snatch	78	3	85	3	91		98	1	104	1	111		117		124		130		137		10				858				4					
4	6	3a	Power Clean	96	3	104	3	112	3	120	1	128	1	136		144		152		160		168		10				1056				4					
4	6	3b	Jerk	96	1	104		112		120	1	128		136		144		152		160		168		4				432									
4	6	4	Romanian Deadlift	96		104		112		120		128		136		144	16	152	16	160		168		16				2304				4					
4	6	5	Press	54		59		63		68		72	20	77		81		86		90		95		20	73	326	1969	1440	8528	38340	230598	4	21	87	475	117.6	117.1142712

WEIGHTLIFTING PROGRAMMING

Table A.1 20-Week Program Excel Analysis: Week 5

Wk	Day	Order	Exercise	60%	R	65%	R	70%	R	75%	R	80%	R	85%	R	90%	R	95%	R	100%	R	105%	R	Vol	Dvol	Wvol	Mvol	Load	Dload	WkLoad	MoLoad	Sets	Dsets	WkSets	MoSets	WkAvl	MAvl
5	1	1	Back Squat	150	5	163	5	175		188	5	200		213		225	12	238		250		263		30				5625				6					
5	1	2	Snatch	78	4	85	4	91	4	98	4	104	4	111	4	117		124		130		137		24				2418				6					
5	1	3a	Clean	96	4	104	4	112	4	120		128	3	136		144		152		160		168		20				2368				5					
5	1	3b	Jerk	78	1	85	1	91	1	98	1	104		111		117		124	16	130		137		5				592									
5	1	4	Snatch High Pull	78		85		91		98		104		111		117	16	124		130		137		16				1872				4					
5	1	5	Press	48		52		56		60		64		68		72	20	76		80		84		20	115			1360	14235			4	25				
5	2	1	Back Squat	150	3	163	3	175	3	188	3	200	3	213	3	225	12	238		250		263		21				4125				7					
5	2	2a	Power Snatch	78	3	85	3	91		98		104		111		117		124		130		137		15				1306.5				5					
5	2	2b	Push Press	78	3	85	3	91		98		104		111		117		124		130		137		15				1306.5				5					
5	2	2c	Overhead Squat	78	3	85	3	91		98		104		111		117		124		130		137		15				1306.5				5					
5	2	3a	Power Clean	96	3	104	3	112	3	120		128		136		144		152		160		168		15				1608				5					
5	2	3b	Front Squat	96	3	104	3	112	3	120		128		136		144		152		160		168		15				1608				5					
5	2	3c	Power Jerk	96	3	104	3	112	3	120		128		136		144		152		160		168		15				1608				5					
5	2	4	Clean Extension	96		104		112		120		128		136		144	16	152		160		168		16				2304				4					
5	2	5	Good Morning	48		52		56		60		64		68		72		76		80	32	84		32	159			2560	17733			4	25				
5	3	1	Front Squat	120	4	130	2	140	4	150		160	12	170		180		190		200		210		20				2960				5					
5	3	2	Snatch	78	2	85	2	91	2	98	2	104	2	111	2	117		124		130		137		8				767				4					
5	3	3a	Clean	96	2	104	2	112	2	120		128	2	136		144		152		160		168		8				944				4					
5	3	3b	Jerk	96	1	104	1	112	1	120	1	128		136		144		152		160		168		4				472									
5	3	4	Romanian Deadlift	96		104		112		120		128		136		144	16	152		160		168		16	56			2304	7447			4	17				
5	4	1	Back Squat	150	5	163	3	175	5	188	5	200	9	213	7	225	6	238		250		263		26				4912.5				6					
5	4	2a	Power Snatch	78	3	85	3	91		98		104		111		117		124		130		137		15				1306.5				5					
5	4	2b	Overhead Squat	78	3	85	3	91		98		104		111		117		124		130		137		15				1306.5				5					
5	4	3a	Power Clean	96	3	104	3	112	3	120		128		136		144		152		160		168		15				1608				5					
5	4	3b	Power Jerk	96	3	104	3	112	3	120		128		136		144		152		160		168		15				1608				5					
5	4	4	Snatch Extension	78		85		91		98		104		111	25	117	25	124		130		137		25				2762.5				5					
5	4	5	Press	48		52		56		60		64		68		72	20	76		80		84		20	131			1440	14944			4	25				
5	5	1	Back Squat	150	3	163	4	175	3	188	3	200	3	213	3	225	6	238		250		263		15				2850				5					
5	5	2	Snatch	78	4	85	4	91	4	98	4	104	4	111	12	117		124		130		137		20				1924				5					
5	5	3a	Clean	96	4	104	4	112	4	120	1	128	12	136	12	144		152		160		168		20				2368				5					
5	5	3b	Jerk	96	1	104	1	112	1	120	3	128	3	136		144		152		160		168		5				592									
5	5	4	Push Press	96	4	104	4	112	4	120	12	128		136		144		152		160		168		20	80			2144	9878			5	20				
5	6	1	Front Squat	120	4	130	4	140	4	150	4	160	4	170	4	180	9	190		200		210		21				3210				6					
5	6	2	Power Snatch	78	4	85	4	91	16	98		104		111		117		124		130		137		24				2106				6					
5	6	3a	Power Clean	96	4	104	4	112	4	120		128		136		144		152		160		168		20				2144				5					
5	6	3b	Jerk	96	1	104	1	112	1	120	3	128		136		144		152		160		168		5				536									
5	6	4	Clean High Pull	96		104		112		120		128		136		144	20	152		160		168		20				2720				5					
5	6	5	Good Morning	48		52		56		60		64		68		72		76		80	32	84		32	122	663		2560	13276	64637.5		4	26	138			97.5

Table A.1 20-Week Program Excel Analysis: Week 6

Wk	Day	Order	Exercise	60%	R	65%	R	70%	R	75%	R	80%	R	85%	R	90%	R	95%	R	100%	R	105%	R	Vol	Dvol	Wvol	Mvol	Load	Dload	WtLoad	MoLoad	Sets	Dsets	Wk-Sets	MoSets	Wk/Avl	MAvl
6	1	1	Snatch	78	4	85		91	4	98		104	16	111		117		124		130		137		24				2340				6					
6	1	2a	Clean	96	4	104		112	4	120		128	12	136		144		152		160		168		20				2368				5					
6	1	2b	Jerk	96	1	104		112	1	120		128	3	136		144		152		160		168		5				592									
6	1	3	Behind Neck Power Jerk	96	3	104	3	112	3	120	3	128		136		144		152		160		168		12				1296				4					
6	1	4	Snatch Extension	78		85		91		98		104	16	111		117		124		130		137		16				1664				8					
6	1	5	Clean Deadlift w/2 halts	96		104		112		120		128		136	12	144		152		160		168		12				1632				4					
6	1	6	Back Squat	150	3	163		175	3	188		200	3	213	2	225		238		250		263		11	100			2000	11892			4	31				
6	2	1	Back Squat	150	4	163		175	4	188		200	16	213		225		238		250		263		24				4500				6					
6	2	2a	Power Snatch	78		85		91		98		104		111		117		124		130		137		13				1111.5				4					
6	2	2b	Overhead Squat	78		85		91		98		104		111		117		124		130		137		12				1033.5									
6	2	3a	Power Clean	96		104		112		120		128		136		144		152		160		168		12				1272				4					
6	2	3b	Power Jerk	96		104		112		120		128		136		144		152		160		168		9				944									
6	2	4	Clean High Pull	96		104		112		120		128		136		144	8	152		160		168		14	84			1944	10805			6	20				
6	3	1	Snatch	78		85		91		98		104		111		117		124		130		137		12				1170				6					
6	3	2a	Clean	96		104		112		120		128		136		144		152		160		168		10				1184				5					
6	3	2b	Jerk	96		104		112		120		128		136		144		152		160		168		7				800									
6	3	4a	Power Clean	96		104		112		120		128		136		144		152		160		168		5				536				5					
6	3	4b	Push Press	96		104		112		120		128		136		144		152		160		168		15				1608									
6	3	5	Good Morning	48		52		56		60		64		68		72		76		80	32	84		32	81			2560	7858			4	20				
6	4	1	Back Squat	150		163		175		188		200		213		225		238		250		263		20				3687.5				7					
6	4	2a	Snatch Extension	78		85		91		98		104		111		117		124		130		137		15				1443				5					
6	4	2b	Snatch	78		85		91		98		104		111		117		124		130		137		5				481									
6	4	3a	Clean	96		104		112		120		128		136		144		152		160		168		5				568				5					
6	4	3b	Front Squat	96		104		112		120		128		136		144		152		160		168		15				1704									
6	4	3c	Jerk	96		104		112		120		128		136		144		152		160		168		5				568									
6	4	4	Snatch Deadlift on blocks	78		85		91		98		104		111		117	16	124		130		137		16				1872				4					
6	4	5	Press	48		52		56		60		64		68		72	20	76		80		84		20	101			1440	11764			4	25				
6	5	1a	Power Snatch	78		85		91		98		104		111		117		124		130		137		12				1033.5				5					
6	5	1b	Push Press	78		85		91		98		104		111		117		124		130		137		15				1306.5				5					
6	5	2	Power Clean	96		104		112		120		128		136		144		152		160		168		17				1808				5					
6	5	3	Clean Extension	96		104		112		120		128	25	136		144		152		160		168		25				3200				5					
6	5	4	Front Squat	120		130		140		150		160		170		180		190		200		210		12	81			1740	9088			4	19				
6	6	1	Back Squat	150		163		175		188		200		213		225		238		250		263		8				1475				4					
6	6	2	Snatch	78		85		91		98		104		111		117		124		130		137		8				767				4					
6	6	3a	Clean Extension	96		104		112		120		128		136		144		152		160		168		15				1704				5					
6	6	3b	Clean	96		104		112		120		128		136		144		152		160		168		5				568				5					
6	6	4	Behind Neck Power Jerk	96		104		112		120		128		136		144		152		160		168		17				1808									
6	6	5	Good Morning	48		52		56		60		64		68		72		76		80	32	84		32	85	532		2560	8882	60288.5		4	22	137		113.3	

Table A.1 20-Week Program Excel Analysis: Week 7

Wk	Day	Order	Exercise	60%	R	65%	R	70%	R	75%	R	80%	R	85%	R	90%	R	95%	R	100%	R	105%	R	Vol	Dvol	Wvol	Mvol	Load	Dload	WkLoad	MoLoad	Sets	Dsets	WkSets	MoSets	WkAvl	MAvl
7	1	1	Snatch	78	2	85		91	2	98		104	4	111	4	117	1	124		130		137		13				1313				7					
7	1	2a	Clean	96	2	104		112	2	120		128	4	136	4	144	1	152		160		168		13				1616				7					
7	1	2b	Jerk	96	1	104		112	1	120		128	2	136	2	144	1	152		160		168		7				880									
7	1	3	Snatch Extension	78		85		91		98		104		111		117		124	15	130		137		15				1852.5				5					
7	1	4	Back Squat	150	3	163		175	3	188		200	3	213		225	9	238		250		263		18				3487.5				6					
7	1		Press	48		52		56		60		64		68		72		76		80		84		16	82			1152	10301			4	29				
7	2	1	Power Snatch	78	3	85		91	6	98	1	104	1	111		117		124		130		137		16				1384.5				6					
7	2	2a	Power Clean	96	3	104		112	6	120	1	128	1	136		144		152		160		168		16				1704				6					
7	2	2b	Jerk	96	1	104		112	2	120	1	128		136		144		152		160		168		6				648									
7	2	3	Clean Extension	96		104		112		120		128		136		144	12	152		160		168		12				1728				4					
7	2	4	Back Squat	150	2	163		175	2	188		200	2	213	2	225	1	238		250		263		9	59			1700	7165			5	21				
7	3	1	Snatch	78	1	85		91	1	98		104	10	111	10	117	1	124		130		137		14				1436.5				8					
7	3	2a	Clean	96	1	104		112	1	120		128	10	136	10	144	1	152		160		168		14				1768				8					
7	3	2b	Jerk	96	1	104		112	1	120		128	4	136	4	144	1	152		160		168		8				1000									
7	3	3	Romanian Deadlift	96		104		112		120		128		136	16	144	16	152		160		168		16	52			2176	6381			4	20				
7	5	1	Power Snatch	78	4	85		91	4	98		104		111		117		124		130		137		20				1742				5					
7	5	2a	Power Clean	96	4	104		112	4	120		128		136		144		152		160		168		20				2144				5					
7	5	2b	Jerk	96	1	104		112	1	120		128		136		144		152		160		168		5				536									
7	5	3a	Front Squat	96		104		112		120		128	8	136	8	144		152		160		168		10				1248				5					
7	5	3b	Jerk	96		104		112	2	120	2	128	8	136	8	144		152		160		168		10				1248									
7	5	4	Front Squat	120		130		140		150		160		170	12	180		190		200		210		12				2040				4					
7	5	5	Press	48		52		56		60		64		68		72		76		80		84		16	93			1152	10110			4	23				
7	6	1	Snatch	78	2	85		91	2	98		104	2	111	2	117	6	124		130		137		12				1209				6					
7	6	2a	Clean	96	2	104		112	2	120		128	2	136	2	144	6	152		160		168		12				1488				6					
7	6	2b	Jerk	96	1	104		112	1	120		128	1	136	1	144	3	152		160		168		6				744									
7	6	3	Romanian Deadlift	96		104		112		120		128		136		144	16	152		160		168		16				2304				4					
7	6	4	Push Press	96	4	104		112	8	120		128		136		144		152		160		168		16	62	348		1696	7441	41397		4	20	113		119.0	

Table A.1 20-Week Program Excel Analysis: Week 7

Table A.1 20-Week Program Excel Analysis: Week 8

Wk	Day	Order	Exercise	60%	R	65%	70%	R	75%	R	80%	R	85%	R	90%	R	95%	R	100%	R	105%	R	Vol	Dvol	Wvol	Mvol	Load	Dload	WkLoad	MoLoad	Sets	Dsets	WkSets	MoSets	WkAvl	MAvl
8	1	1	Snatch	78	1	85	91	1	98	1	104	1	111	1	117	3	124	3	130	3	137		12				1326				12					
8	1	2a	Clean	96	1	104	112	1	120	1	128	1	136	1	144	3	152	3	160	3	168		12				1632				12					
8	1	2b	Jerk	96	1	104	112	1	120	1	128	1	136	1	144	3	152	3	160	3	168		12				1632				12					
8	1	3	Front Squat	120	1	130	140	1	150	1	160	1	170	1	180	3	190	3	200	3	210		12				2040				12					
8	1	4	Snatch Extension	78		85	91		98		104		111		117		124		130	12	137		12				1482				4					
8	1	5	Press	48		52	56		60		64		68		72	16	76		80		84		16	76			1152	9264			4	44				
8	2	1	Snatch	78	2	85	91	2	98	2	104	2	111	2	117	4	124		130		137		10				988				6					
8	2	2a	Clean	96	2	104	112	2	120	2	128	2	136	2	144	2	152		160		168		8				944				4					
8	2	2b	Jerk	96	1	104	112	1	120	1	128	1	136	1	144	1	152		160		168		4				472									
8	2	3	Clean Extension	96		104	112		120		128		136		144	12	152		160		168		12				1728				4					
8	2	4	Back Squat	150	3	163	175	3	188	3	200	3	213	3	225	6	238		250		263		15	49			2850	6982			5	19				
8	3	1	Power Snatch	78	1	85	91	3	98	3	104	3	111		117		124		130		137		10				897				10					
8	3	2a	Power clean	96	1	104	112	3	120	3	128	3	136		144		152		160		168		10				1104				10					
8	3	2b	Jerk	96	1	104	112	3	120	3	128	3	136		144		152		160		168		10				1104				5					
8	3	4	Push Press	96	3	104	112	3	120	6	128		136		144		152		160		168		12				1272				5					
8	3	5	Good Morning	48		52	56		60		64		68		72		76		80	16	84		16	58			1280	5657			4	29				
8	5	1	Snatch	78	2	85	91	2	98	2	104	2	111	2	117	4	124		130		137		10				988				6					
8	5	2a	Clean	96	2	104	112	2	120	2	128	2	136	2	144	2	152		160		168		8				944				4					
8	5	2b	Jerk	96	1	104	112	1	120	1	128	1	136	1	144	1	152		160		168		4				472									
8	5	3	Front Squat	120	3	130	140	3	150	3	160	3	170	3	180	3	190	3	200	3	210		15				2310				7					
8	5	4	Press	48		52	56		60		64		68		72	16	76		80		84		16	53			1152	5666			4	21				
8	6	1	Snatch	78	2	85	91	2	98	2	104	2	111	2	117	2	124		130		137		8				767				4					
8	6	2a	Clean	96	2	104	112	2	120	2	128	2	136	2	144	2	152		160		168		8				944				4					
8	6	2b	Jerk	96	1	104	112	1	120	1	128	1	136	1	144	1	152		160		168		4				472									
8	6	3	Snatch Extension	78		85	91		98		104		111		117	12	124	12	130		137		12				1404				4					
8	6	4	Clean Extension	96		104	112		120		128		136	9	144	9	152		160	9	168		9	41	277	1820	1224	4811	32580	198903	4	16	129	517	117.6	109.2873626

WEIGHTLIFTING PROGRAMMING

Wk	Day	Order	Exercise	60%	R	65%	R	70%	R	75%	R	80%	R	85%	R	90%	R	95%	R	100%	R	105%	R	Vol	Dvol	Wvol	Mvol	Load	Dload	WkLoad	MoLoad	Sets	Dsets	WkSets	MoSets	WkAvl	MAvl
9	1	1	Snatch	78	1	85	1	91	1	98	1	104	1	111	1	117	1	124		130		137		4				383.5				4					
9	1	2a	Clean	96	1	104	1	112	1	120	1	128	1	136	1	144	1	152		160		168		4				472				4					
9	1	2b	Jerk	96	1	104	1	112	1	120	1	128	1	136	1	144	1	152		160		168		4				472				4					
9	1	3	Front Squat	120	2	130	2	140	2	150	2	160	2	170	2	180	2	190		200		210		8				1180				4					
9	1	4	Press	48		52		56		60		64		68		72	16	76		80		84		16	36			1152	3660			4	16				
9	2	1	Power Snatch	78	2	85	2	91	6	98	6	104		111		117		124		130		137		8				702				4					
9	2	2a	Power Clean	96	2	104	2	112	6	120	6	128		136		144		152		160		168		8				864				4					
9	2	2b	Jerk	96	1	104	1	112	3	120	3	128		136		144		152		160		168		4				432				4					
9	2	3	Back Squat	150	3	163	3	175	9	188	9	200		213		225		238		250		263		12	32			2025	4023			4	12				
9	4	1	Power Snatch	78	6	85	6	91		98		104		111		117		124		130		137		6				468				3					
9	4	2a	Power Clean	96	6	104	6	112		120		128		136		144		152		160		168		6				576				3					
9	4	2b	Jerk	96	3	104	3	112		120		128		136		144		152		160		168		3				288				3					
9	4	3	Front Squat	120	3	130	3	140	6	150	6	160		170		180		190		200		210		9	24	72		1200	2532	7707		3	9	37		107.0	

Table A.1 20-Week Program Excel Analysis: Week 9

Table A.1 20-Week Program Excel Analysis: Week 10

Wk	Day	Order	Exercise	60%	R	65%	R	70%	R	75%	R	80%	R	85%	R	90%	R	95%	R	100%	R	105%	R	Vol	Dvol	Wvol	Mvol	Load	Dload	WktLoad	MoLoad	Sets	Dsets	WkSets	MoSets	WkAvl	MAvl
10	1	1	Back Squat	150	4	163	4	175	4	188		200	12	213		225	2	238	1	250		263		20				3700				5					
10	1	2	Power Snatch	78	4	85	4	91	9	98	9	104		111		117		124		130		137		17				1469				5					
10	1	3a	Power Clean	96	4	104	4	112	9	120	9	128		136		144		152		160		168		17				1808				5					
10	1	3b	Jerk	96	1	104	1	112	3	120	3	128		136		144		152		160		168		5				536									
10	1	4	Romanian Deadlift	96	4	104	4	112	9	120	9	128	20	136		144		152		160		168		20				2560				4					
10	1	5	Push Press	96	4	104	4	112	9	120	9	128		136		144		152		160		168		17	96			1808	11381			5	24				
10	2	1	Back Squat	150	3	163	3	175	3	188	3	200	3	213	2	225	2	238	1	250		263		12				2225				5					
10	2	2	Snatch	78	3	85	3	91	3	98	3	104	12	111		117		124		130		137		18				1755				6					
10	2	3a	Clean	96	3	104	3	112	3	120	3	128	9	136		144		152		160		168		15				1776				5					
10	2	3b	Jerk	96	1	104	1	112	1	120	1	128	3	136	3	144		152		160		168		5				592									
10	2	4	Snatch Deadlift	78	1	85	1	91		98		104		111		117		124	20	130		137		20				2340				5					
10	2	5	Hang Snatch High Pull	78		85		91		98		104		111		117	12	124	12	130		137		12		82		1404	10092			4	25				
10	3	1	Front Squat	120	4	130	4	140	4	150	4	160	12	170	12	180		190		200		210		20				2960				5					
10	3	2	Snatch	78	2	85	2	91	2	98	2	104	4	111	4	117		124		130		137		8				754				4					
10	3	3a	Clean	96	2	104	2	112	2	120	2	128	4	136	4	144		152		160		168		8				928				4					
10	3	3b	Jerk	96	1	104	1	112	1	120	1	128	2	136	2	144		152		160		168		4				464									
10	3	4	Clean Extension	96		104		112		120		128		136	12	144	12	152		160		168		12		52		1632	6738			4	17				
10	4	1	Back Squat	150	3	163	3	175	3	188	3	200	3	213	3	225	12	238		250		263		21				4125				7					
10	4	2a	Power Snatch	78	3	85	3	91	6	98	6	104		111		117		124		130		137		12				1033.5				5					
10	4	2b	Overhead Squat	78	3	85	3	91	9	98	9	104		111		117		124		130		137		15				1306.5									
10	4	3a	Power Clean	96	3	104	3	112	6	120	6	128		136		144		152		160		168		12				1272				5					
10	4	3b	Jerk	96	2	104	2	112	6	120	6	128		136		144		152		160		168		10				1072									
10	4	4	Romanian Deadlift	96		104		112		120		128		136		144	20	152	20	160		168		20				2720				4					
10	4	5	Press	48		52		56		60		64		68		72	16	76	16	80		84		16	106			1152	12681			4	25				
10	5	1	Front Squat	120	3	130	3	140	3	150	3	160	6	170	6	180	5	190	1	200		210		18				2770				7					
10	5	2	Snatch	78	2	85	2	91	2	98	2	104	2	111	2	117	4	124		130		137		10				988				5					
10	5	3a	Clean	96	2	104	2	112	2	120	2	128	2	136	2	144	4	152		160		168		10				1216				5					
10	5	3b	Jerk	96	1	104	1	112	1	120	1	128	1	136	1	144	2	152		160		168		5				608									
10	5	4	Snatch Extension	78		85		91		98		104		111		117	15	124	15	130		137		15		58		1755	7337			5	22				
10	6	1	Back Squat	150	4	163	4	175	4	188	4	200	8	213		225		238		250		263		16				2900				4					
10	6	2	Power Snatch	78	4	85	4	91	9	98	9	104		111		117		124		130		137		17				1469				5					
10	6	3a	Power Clean	96	4	104	4	112	9	120	9	128		136		144		152		160		168		17				1808				5					
10	6	3b	Jerk	96	2	104	2	112	3	120	3	128		136		144		152		160		168		7				736									
10	6	4	Clean High Pull	96		104		112		120		128	16	136	16	144		152		160		168		16				2048				4					
10	6	5	Press	48		52		56		60		64		68		72	20	76	20	80		84		20	93	487		1440	10401	59130		4	22	135			121.4

Table A.1 20-Week Program Excel Analysis: Week 11

Wk	Day	Order	Exercise	60%	R	65%	R	70%	R	75%	R	80%	R	85%	R	90%	R	95%	R	100%	R	105%	R	Vol	Dvol	Vvol	Mvol	Load	Dload	WkLoad	MoLoad	Sets	Dsets	WkSets	MoSets	WkAvl	MAvl
11	1	1	Back Squat	150		163		175		188		200		213		225		238		250		263		25				4625				5					
11	1	2	Snatch	78		85		91		98		104		111		117		124		130		137		19				1839.5				5					
11	1	3a	Clean	96		104		112		120		128		136		144		152		160		168		19				2264				5					
11	1	3b	Jerk	96		104		112		120		128		136		144		152		160		168		5				600									
11	1	4	Snatch High Pull	78		85		91		98		104		111		117		124		130		137		16				1768				4					
11	1	5	Good Morning	48		52		56		60		64		68		72		76		80		84		24	108			1920	13017			4	23				
11	2	1	Back Squat	150		163		175		188		200		213		225		238		250		263		15				2775				5					
11	2	2a	Power Snatch	78		85		91		98		104		111		117		124		130		137		12				1033.5				5					
11	2	2b	Push Press	78		85		91		98		104		111		117		124		130		137		12				1033.5									
11	2	2c	Overhead Squat	78		85		91		98		104		111		117		124		130		137		12				1033.5									
11	2	3a	Power Clean	96		104		112		120		128		136		144		152		160		168		12				1272				5					
11	2	3b	Front Squat	96		104		112		120		128		136		144		152		160		168		12				1272									
11	2	3c	Jerk	96		104		112		120		128		136		144		152		160		168		12				1272									
11	2	4	Romanian Deadlift	96		104		112		120		128		136		144		152		160		168		16				2176				4					
11	2	5	Press	48		52		56		60		64		68		72		76		80		84		12	127			912	12780			4	23				
11	3	1	Back Squat	150		163		175		188		200		213		225		238		250		263		12				2212.5				4					
11	3	2	Snatch	78		85		91		98		104		111		117		124		130		137		8				767				4					
11	3	3a	Clean	96		104		112		120		128		136		144		152		160		168		8				944				4					
11	3	3b	Jerk	96		104		112		120		128		136		144		152		160		168		4				472									
11	3	4	Snatch Extension	78		85		91		98		104		111		117		124		130		137		8	40			884	5280			4	16				
11	4	1	Front Squat	120		130		140		150		160		170		180		190		200		210		25				3700				5					
11	4	2	Snatch	78		85		91		98		104		111		117		124		130		137		20				1924				5					
11	4	3a	Clean	96		104		112		120		128		136		144		152		160		168		20				2368				5					
11	4	3b	Jerk	96		104		112		120		128		136		144		152		160		168		5				592									
11	4	4	Romanian Deadlift	96		104		112		120		128		136		144		152		160		168		20				2720				4					
11	4	5	Press	48		52		56		60		64		68		72		76		80		84		12	102			912	12216			4	23				
11	5	1	Back Squat	150		163		175		188		200		213		225		238		250		263		18				3375				6					
11	5	2	Power Snatch	78		85		91		98		104		111		117		124		130		137		20				1742				5					
11	5	3a	Power Clean	96		104		112		120		128		136		144		152		160		168		20				2144				5					
11	5	3b	Jerk	96		104		112		120		128		136		144		152		160		168		5				536									
11	5	4	Clean Extension	96		104		112		120		128		136		144		152		160		168		20				2720				5					
11	5	5	Good Morning	48		52		56		60		64		68		72		76		80		84		32	115			2560	13077			4	25				
11	6	1	Back Squat	150		163		175		188		200		213		225		238		250		263		16				2950				4					
11	6	2	Snatch	78		85		91		98		104		111		117		124		130		137		8				767				4					
11	6	3a	Clean	96		104		112		120		128		136		144		152		160		168		8				944				4					
11	6	3b	Jerk	96		104		112		120		128		136		144		152		160		168		4				472									
11	6	4	Push Press	96		104		112		120		128		136		144		152		160		168		17				1808				5					
11	6	5	Hang Snatch High Pull	78		85		91		98		104		111		117		124		130		137		16	69	561		1664	8605	64973.5		4	21	131			115.8

Wk	Day	Order	Exercise	60%	R	65%	R	70%	R	75%	R	80%	R	85%	R	90%	R	95%	R	100%	R	105%	R	Vol	Dvol	Wvol	Mvol	Load	Dload	WkLoad	MoLoad	Sets	Dsets	WkSets	MoSets	WkAvl	MAvl
12	1	1	Back Squat	150	4	163		175	4	188	4	200	4	213		225	12	238		250		263		28				5500				7					
12	1	2	Snatch	78	3	85	3	91	3	98		104		111		117	12	124		130		137		21				2145				7					
12	1	3a	Clean	96	3	104	3	112	3	120		128		136		144	9	152		160		168		18				2232				6					
12	1	3b	Jerk	96	1	104	1	112	1	120		128		136		144	3	152		160		168		6				744									
12	1	4	Power Jerk	96	4	104	4	112	12	120		128		136		144		152		160		168		20	93			2144	12765			5	25				
12	2	1	Back Squat	150	2	163		175	2	188	2	200		213	2	225	2	238	2	250		263		12				2375				5					
12	2	2	Snatch	78	2	85	2	91	2	98	2	104		111		117	1	124		130		137		9				884				5					
12	2	3a	Clean	96	2	104	2	112	2	120	2	128		136		144	1	152		160		168		9				1088				5					
12	2	3b	Jerk	96	1	104	1	112		120	1	128	1	136		144	1	152		160		168		5				616									
12	2	4	Snatch High Pull	78		85		91		98		104		111		117	15	124		130		137		15	50			1755	6718			5	20				
12	4	1	Back Squat	150	4	163		175	4	188		200	8	213		225		238		250		263		16				2900				4					
12	4	2	Power Snatch	78	3	85	3	91	9	98		104		111		117		124		130		137		15				1306.5				5					
12	4	3a	Power Clean	96	3	104	3	112	9	120		128		136		144		152		160		168		15				1608				5					
12	4	3b	Jerk	96	1	104	1	112	3	120		128		136		144		152		160		168		5				536									
12	4	4	Clean Extension	96		104		112		120		128		136		144	15	152		160		168		15				2160				5					
12	4	5	Press	48		52		56		60		64		68	20	72		76		80		84		20	86			1360	9871			4	23				
12	5	1	Front Squat	120	4	130		140	4	150	4	160	4	170		180	8	190		200		210		24				3720				6					
12	5	2	Snatch	78	2	85	2	91	2	98	2	104	2	111	2	117	2	124		130		137		14				1430				7					
12	5	3a	Clean	96	2	104	2	112	2	120	2	128	2	136	2	144		152		160		168		12				1488				7					
12	5	3b	Jerk	96	1	104	1	112	1	120	1	128	1	136		144	1	152		160		168		6				744									
12	5	4	Good Morning	48		52		56		60		64		68		72		76		80	24	84		24	80			1920	9302			4	24				
12	6	1	Back Squat	150	2	163		175	2	188	2	200	2	213	2	225		238		250		263		10				1850				5					
12	6	2	Snatch Extension	78		85		91		98		104		111		117	20	124		130		137		20				2340				5					
12	6	3	Clean Extension	96		104		112		120		128		136		144	20	152		160		168		20				2720				5					
12	6	4	Press	48		52		56		60		64		68		72	16	76		80		84		16	66	375	1495	1152	8062	46717.5	178528	4	19	111	414	124.6	119.4167224

Table A.1 20-Week Program Excel Analysis: Week 12

WEIGHTLIFTING PROGRAMMING

Table A.1 20-Week Program Excel Analysis: Week 13

Wk	Day	Order	Exercise	60%	R	65%	R	70%	R	75%	R	80%	R	85%	R	90%	R	95%	R	100%	R	105%	R	Vol	Dvol	Wvol	Mvol	Load	Dload	WkLoad	MoLoad	Sets	Dsets	WkSets	MoSets	WkAvl	MAvl
13	1	1	Back Squat	150		163	4	175	4	188	4	200	4	213	4	225	12	238		250		263		24				4650				6					
13	1	2	Snatch	78		85	4	91	4	98	4	104	4	111	4	117	9	124		130		137		21				2086.5				6					
13	1	3a	Clean	96		104	4	112	4	120	4	128	4	136	4	144	9	152		160		168		21				2568				6					
13	1	3b	Jerk	96		104	1	112	1	120	1	128	1	136	1	144	3	152		160		168		6				744									
13	1	4	Snatch Extension	78		85	1	91	1	98	1	104	1	111	1	117		124	16	130		137		16				1872				4					
13	1	5	Press	48		52		56		60		64		68		72	20	76		80		84		20	108			1360	13281			4	26				
13	2	1	Back Squat	150		163	3	175	3	188	3	200	3	213	3	225	3	238		250		263		12				2212.5				4					
13	2	2a	Power Snatch	78		85	3	91	9	98	9	104		111		117		124		130		137		15				1306.5				5					
13	2	2b	Push Press	78		85	3	91	9	98	9	104		111		117		124		130		137		15				1306.5				5					
13	2	2c	Overhead Squat	78		85	3	91	9	98	9	104		111		117		124		130		137		15				1306.5				5					
13	2	3a	Power Clean	96		104	3	112	3	120	9	128		136		144		152		160		168		15				1608				5					
13	2	3b	Front Squat	96		104	3	112	3	120	9	128		136		144		152		160		168		15				1608				5					
13	2	3c	Jerk	96		104	3	112	3	120	9	128		136		144		152		160		168		15				1608				5					
13	2	4	Clean Extension	96		104		112		120		128		136	16	144	16	152		160		168		16	118			2176	13132			4	18				
13	3	1	Front Squat	120		130	4	140	4	150	4	160	4	170	4	180	9	190		200		210		21				3210				6					
13	3	2	Snatch	78		85	2	91	2	98	2	104	2	111	2	117	2	124		130		137		8				767				4					
13	3	3a	Clean	96		104	2	112	2	120	2	128	2	136	2	144	2	152		160		168		8				944				4					
13	3	3b	Jerk	96		104	1	112	1	120	1	128	1	136	1	144	1	152		160		168		4				472									
13	3	4	Romanian Deadlift	96		104		112	4	120		128		136		144	20	152	20	160		168		20				2880				4					
13	3	5	Push Press	96		104	4	112	9	120		128		136		144		152		160		168		17	78			1808	10081			4	22				
13	4	1	Back Squat	150		163	4	175	4	188	4	200	4	213	4	225	9	238		250		263		21				4012.5				6					
13	4	2	Power Snatch	78		85	4	91	16	98	16	104		111		117		124		130		137		24				2106				6					
13	4	3a	Power Clean	96		104	4	112	16	120	16	128		136		144		152		160		168		24				2592				6					
13	4	3b	Jerk	96		104	1	112	4	120	4	128		136		144		152		160		168		6				648									
13	4	4	Snatch High Pull	78		85		91		98		104		111		117	15	124	15	130		137		15				1755				4					
13	4	5	Press	48		52		56		60		64		68		72	20	76		80		84		20	110			1360	12474			4	26				
13	5	1	Back Squat	150		163	4	175	4	188	4	200	4	213	4	225	3	238		250		263		15				2737.5				4					
13	5	2	Snatch	78		85	3	91	3	98	3	104	3	111	3	117	3	124		130		137		12				1150.5				4					
13	5	3a	Clean	96		104	3	112	4	120	4	128	3	136		144		152		160		168		12				1416				4					
13	5	3b	Jerk	96		104	1	112	1	120	1	128	1	136	1	144	1	152		160		168		4				472									
13	5	4	Clean High Pull	96		104		112		120		128		136		144	16	152	16	160		168		16				2304				4					
13	5	5	Good Morning	48		52		56		60		64		68		72	32	76		80	32	84		32	91			2560	10640			4	20				
13	6	1	Back Squat	150		163	3	175	3	188	3	200	9	213	9	225		238		250		263		15				2775				6					
13	6	2	Power Snatch	78		85	4	91	4	98	4	104	3	111	3	117	3	124		130		137		16				1352				4					
13	6	3a	Power Clean	96		104	4	112	4	120	4	128	4	136		144		152		160		168		16				1664				4					
13	6	3b	Jerk	96		104	2	112	2	120		128		136		144		152		160		168		4				416									
13	6	4	Romanian Deadlift	96		104		112		120		128		136		144	20	152		160		168		20	71	576		2880	9087	68694		4	18	130		119.3	

Table A.1 (continued)

Wk	Day	Order	Exercise	60%	R	65%	R	70%	R	75%	R	80%	R	85%	R	90%	R	95%	R	100%	R	105%	R	Vol	Dvol	Wvol	Mvol	Load	Dload	WkLoad	MoLoad	Sets	Dsets	WkSets	MoSets	WkAvl	MAvl
14	1	1	1 Snatch	78	1	85		91	1	98	1	104	10	111	1	117	1	124	1	130		137	1	14				1436.5				8					
14	1	2a	Clean	96	1	104		112	1	120	1	128	10	136	1	144	1	152	1	160		168	1	14				1768				8					
14	1	2b	Jerk	96	1	104	1	112	1	120	1	128	4	136	4	144		152	12	160		168		8				1000				4					
14	1		3 Snatch Extension	78		85		91	3	98	9	104		111		117		124		130		137		12				1404				4					
14	1		4 Power Jerk	96	3	104	3	112	3	120	9	128		136		144		152		160		168		15				1608				5					
14	1		5 Back Squat	150	3	163	3	175	3	188	3	200	12	213	3	225	3	238	1	250		263		22	85			4237.5	11454			8	33				
14	2	1	Power Snatch	78	1	85	1	91	1	98	10	104		111		117		124		130		137		13				1170				8					
14	2	2a	Power Clean	96	1	104	1	112	1	120	10	128		136		144		152		160		168		13				1440				8					
14	2	2b	Jerk	96	1	104	1	112	3	120	1	128	1	136		144		152		160		168		6				656									
14	2		3 Clean Extension	96		104		112		120		128		136	15	144		152		160		168		15				2040				5	26				
14	2		4 Back Squat	150	2	163		175		188	2	200	2	213	2	225	2	238	1	250		263		9	56			1700	7006			5	26				
14	3	1	Snatch	78	2	85	2	91	2	98	2	104	2	111	2	117	2	124		130		137		8				767				4					
14	3	2a	Clean	96	2	104	2	112	1	120	2	128	2	136	2	144	2	152		160		168		8				944				4					
14	3	2b	Jerk	96	3	104		112	1	120	1	128	1	136	1	144	1	152	1	160		168		4				472				6	14				
14	3		3 Front Squat	120	3	130		140	3	150	3	160	9	170	2	180	9	190	1	200		210		18	38			2790	4973			6	14				
14	4	1	Snatch	78	1	85		91	1	98	1	104	10	111	1	117	1	124	1	130		137	1	14				1436.5				8					
14	4	2a	Clean	96	1	104	1	112	1	120		128	10	136	1	144	1	152	1	160		168		14				1768				8					
14	4	2b	Jerk	96	1	104	1	112	1	120	1	128	4	136	4	144		152	15	160		168		8				1000				5					
14	4		3 Snatch Extension	78		85		91		98	1	104	10	111		117		124		130		137		15				1755				8					
14	4		4 Back Squat	150	1	163		175	1	188		200	10	213	10	225	20	238	1	250		263		14				2762.5				4	33				
14	4		5 Press	48		52		56		60		64		68		72		76		80		84		20	85			1360	10082			5	33				
14	5	1	Snatch	78	1	85		91	1	98	1	104	1	111	1	117	1	124	1	130		137	1	6				611				5					
14	5	2a	Clean	96	1	104	1	112	1	120	1	128	1	136	1	144	1	152	1	160		168		6				752				5					
14	5	2b	Jerk	96	1	104	1	112	1	120	1	128	1	136	1	144	1	152	1	160		168		5	17			616	1979				10				
14	6	1	Power Snatch	78	3	85	3	91	9	98		104		111		117		124		130		137		15				1306.5				5					
14	6	2a	Power	96	3	104	3	112	9	120		128		136		144		152		160		168		15				1608				5					
14	6	2b	Jerk	96	1	104	1	112	3	120		128		136		144		152		160		168		5				536									
14	6		3 Clean Extension	96		104		112		120		128	12	136		144		152		160		168		16				2208				8					
14	6		4 Front Squat	120	1	130		140	1	150	1	160	10	170	1	180	1	190		200		210		13				2030				7					
14	6		5 Good Morning	48		52		56		60		64	10	68		72	1	76		80	24	84		24	88	369		1920	9609	45102.5		4	29	145			122.2

Table A.1 20-Week Program Excel Analysis: Week 14

Wk	Day	Order	Exercise	60%	R	65%	R	70%	R	75%	R	80%	R	85%	R	90%	R	95%	R	100%	R	105%	R	Vol	Dvol	Wvol	Invol	Load	Dload	Wkload	Moload	Sets	Dsets	WkSets	MoSets	WkAvl	MAvl
15	1	1	Snatch	78	1	85	1	91	1	98	1	104	10	111	1	117	2	124		130		137	15				1553.5				9					
15	1	2a	Clean	96	1	104	1	112	1	120	10	128	10	136	2	144	2	152		160		168	15				1912				9					
15	1	2b	Jerk	96	1	104	1	112	1	120	4	128	1	136	2	144	2	152		160		168	9				1144									
15	1	3	Snatch Extension	78		85		91		98		104	6	111		117		124	15	130	15	137	15				1852.5				5					
15	1	4	Front Squat	120	3	130	3	140	3	150	3	160	6	170	4	180	1	190		200		210	17	71			2600	9062			7	30				
15	2	1	Power Snatch	78	1	85	1	91	10	98	2	104		111		117	1	124		130		137	14				1267.5				8					
15	2	2a	Power Clean	96	1	104	1	112	10	120	2	128		136		144	1	152		160		168	14				1560				8					
15	2	2b	Jerk	96	1	104	1	112	4	120	2	128		136		144	1	152		160		168	8				888				8					
15	2	3	Clean Extension	96		104		112		120		128	12	136		144	12	152		160		168	12				1728				4					
15	2	4	Back Squat	150	2	163	2	175	2	188	2	200	2	213	2	225	2	238	2	250		263	10	58			1925	7369			5	25				
15	3	1	Snatch	78	1	85	1	91	1	98	1	104	1	111	1	117	1	124	1	130		137	5				500.5				5					
15	3	2a	Clean	96	1	104	1	112	1	120	1	128	1	136	1	144	1	152	1	160		168	5				616				5					
15	3	2b	Jerk	96	1	104	1	112	1	120	1	128	1	136	1	144	1	152	1	160		168	5				616				5					
15	3	3	Snatch Extension	78		85		91		98		104		111		117	12	124		130		137	12				1404				4					
15	3	4	Front Squat	120	3	130	3	140	3	150	3	160	6	170	4	180	4	190	1	200		210	17	44			2600	5737			5	19				
15	4	1	Power Snatch	78	1	85	1	91	4	98	4	104	1	111		117	1	124		130		137	6				526.5				4					
15	4	2a	Power Clean	96	2	104	2	112	4	120	2	128		136		144		152		160		168	8				848				4					
15	4	2b	Jerk	96	1	104	1	112	1	120	2	128		136		144		152		160		168	4				424				4					
15	4	3	Clean Extension	96		104		112		120		128		136	12	144		152		160		168	12	30	203		1632	3431	25597.5		4	12	86			126.1

Table A.1 20-Week Program Excel Analysis: Week 15

Wk	Day	Order	Exercise	60%	R	65%	R	70%	R	75%	R	80%	R	85%	R	90%	R	95%	R	100%	R	105%	R	Vol	Dvol	Wvol	Mvol	Load	Dload	WkLoad	MoLoad	Sets	Dsets	WkSets	MoSets	WkAvl	MAvl
16	1	1	Snatch	78	1	85	1	91	1	98	1	104	1	111	1	117	1	124	3	130		137		16				1670.5				10					
16	1	2a	Clean	96	1	104	1	112	1	120	1	128	10	136	10	144	1	152	3	160		168		16				2056				10					
16	1	2b	Jerk	96	1	104	1	112	1	120	1	128	4	136	4	144	3	152	3	160		168		10				1288				4					
16	1	3	Snatch Extension	78		85		91		98		104		111		117		124		130	12	137		12				1560				4					
16	1	4	Front Squat	120	1	130	1	140	1	150	1	160	10	170	10	180	1	190	3	200		210		16				2570				10					
16	1	5	Press	48		52		56		60		64		68		72	20	76	20	80		84		20	90			1440	10585			4	38				
16	2	1	Snatch	78	2	85		91	2	98	2	104	8	111	8	117		124		130		137		12				1170				6					
16	2	2a	Clean	96	2	104	2	112	2	120	2	128	2	136	8	144		152		160		168		12				1440				6					
16	2	2b	Jerk	96	1	104	1	112	1	120	1	128	4	136	4	144		152		160		168		6				720									
16	2	3	Clean Extension	96		104		112		120		128		136		144	12	152	12	160		168		12				1728				4					
16	2	4	Front Squat	120	3	130	3	140	3	150	3	160	9	170	9	180		190		200		210		15	57			2220	7278			5	21				
16	3	1	Power Snatch	78	1	85	1	91	10	98	1	104	1	111		117		124		130		137		13				1170				7					
16	3	2a	Power Clean	96	1	104	1	112	10	120	1	128	1	136		144		152		160		168		13				1440				7					
16	3	2b	Jerk	96	1	104	1	112	4	120	1	128	1	136		144		152		160		168		7				768									
16	3	3	Back Squat	150	3	163	3	175	3	188	3	200	3	213	3	225	3	238	1	250		263		13	46			2437.5	5816			5	19				
16	5	1	Snatch	78	1	85	1	91	1	98	1	104	2	111	2	117	2	124	1	130		137		7				715				7					
16	5	2a	Clean	96	1	104	1	112	1	120	1	128	2	136	2	144	2	152	1	160		168		7				880				7					
16	5	2b	Jerk	96	1	104	1	112	1	120	1	128	2	136	2	144	2	152	1	160		168		7				880									
16	5	3	Snatch Extension	78		85		91		98		104		111		117		124		130	15	137		15				1950				5					
16	5	4	Front Squat	120	2	130	2	140	2	150	2	160	4	170	4	180	2	190	2	200		210		14				2200				7					
16	5	5	Press	48		52		56		60		64		68		72	20	76	20	80		84		20	70			1440	8065			4	30				
16	6	1	Power Snatch	78	2	85	2	91	4	98	4	104		111		117		124		130		137		10				858				5					
16	6	2a	Power Clean	96	2	104	4	112	4	120	4	128		136		144		152		160		168		10				1056				5					
16	6	2b	Jerk	96	1	104	1	112	2	120	2	128		136		144		152		160		168		5				528									
16	6	3	Clean Extension	96		104		112		120		128		136		144	12	152	12	160		168		12				1728				4					
16	6	4	Back Squat	150	3	163	3	175	3	188	3	200	3	213	3	225	9	238	3	250	3	263		24				4875				12					
16	6	5	Good Morning	48		52		56		60		64		68		72		76		80	24	84		24	278	541	1689	1920	33564	65306.5	204700.5	4	19	127	488	120.7	121.19627

Table A.1 20-Week Program Excel Analysis: Week 16

Table A.1 20-Week Program Excel Analysis: Week 17

Wk	Day	Order	Exercise	60%	R	65%	R	70%	R	75%	R	80%	R	85%	R	90%	R	95%	R	100%	R	105%	R	Vol	Dvol	Wvol	Mvol	Load	Dload	WkLoad	MoLoad	Sets	Dsets	WkSets	MoSets	WkAvl	MAvl
17	1	1	Snatch	78	1	85	1	91	1	98	1	104	1	111	1	117	3	124	3	130	3	137		12				1326				12	12				
17	1	2a	Clean	96	1	104	1	112	1	120	1	128	1	136	1	144	3	152	3	160	3	168		12				1632				12	12				
17	1	2b	Jerk	96	1	104	1	112	1	120	1	128	1	136	1	144	3	152	3	160	3	168		12				1632				12					
17	1	3	Snatch Extension	78		85		91		98		104		111		117		124		130	15	137		15				1852.5				5					
17	1	4	Front Squat	120	1	130	1	140	1	150	1	160	1	170	1	180	3	190	3	200	3	210		12				2040				12					
17	1	5	Press	48		52		56		60		64		68		72	20	76		80		84		20	83			1440	9923			4	45				
17	2	1	Snatch	78	2	85	2	91	2	98	2	104	2	111	2	117	2	124		130		137		8				767				4					
17	2	2a	Clean	96	2	104	2	112	2	120	2	128	2	136	2	144	2	152		160		168		8				944				4					
17	2	2b	Jerk	96	1	104	1	112	1	120	1	128	1	136	1	144	1	152		160		168		4				472				4					
17	2	3	Clean Extension	96		104		112		120		128		136		144		152	15	160		168		15				2160				5					
17	2	4	Front Squat	120	2	130	2	140	2	150	2	160	4	170	4	180	2	190	2	200	2	210		10	45			1500	5843			5	18				
17	3	1	Power Snatch	78	1	85	1	91	3	98	3	104	3	111		117		124		130		137		10				897				10					
17	3	2a	Power Clean	96	1	104	1	112	3	120	3	128	3	136		144		152		160		168		10				1104				10					
17	3	2b	Jerk	96	1	104	1	112	3	120	3	128	3	136		144		152		160		168		10				1104									
17	3	3	Power Jerk	96	3	104	3	112	9	120	9	128		136		144		152		160		168		15				1608				5					
17	3	4	Back Squat	150	2	163	2	175	2	188	2	200	2	213	2	225	2	238	1	250		263		9	54			1700	6413			5	30				
17	5	1	Snatch	78	1	85	1	91	1	98	1	104	1	111	1	117	3	124	3	130	3	137		12				1326				12					
17	5	2a	Clean	96	1	104	1	112	1	120	1	128	1	136	1	144	3	152	3	160	3	168		12				1632				12					
17	5	2b	Jerk	96	1	104	1	112	1	120	1	128	1	136	1	144	3	152	3	160	3	168		12				1632									
17	5	3	Snatch High Pull	78		85		91		98		104		111		117		124	15	130		137		15				1755				5					
17	5	4	Front Squat	120	2	130	2	140	2	150	2	160	2	170	2	180	2	190	2	200	1	210		11				1730				6					
17	5	5	Good Morning	48		52		56		60		64		68		72		76		80	16	84	16	16	78			1280	9355			4	39				
17	6	1	Power Snatch	78	2	85	2	91	6	98	6	104	6	111		117		124		130		137		10				871				5					
17	6	2a	Power Clean	96	2	104	2	112	6	120	6	128	6	136		144		152		160		168		10				1072				5					
17	6	2b	Jerk	96	1	104	1	112	1	120	3	128		136		144		152		160		168		5				536									
17	6	3a	Front Squat	96		104		112		120		128	8	136	8	144		152		160		168		8				1024				4					
17	6	3b	Jerk	96		104		112		120		128	8	136	8	144		152		160		168		8				1024									
17	6	4	Back Squat	150	3	163	3	175	3	188	3	200	6	213	6	225	5	238	2	250		263		19				3687.5				7					
17	6	5	Press	48		52		56		60		64		68		72		76		80		84		20	80		340	1440	9655	41188		4	25	157			121.1

WEIGHTLIFTING PROGRAMMING

Wk	Day	Order	Exercise	60%	R	65%	R	70%	R	75%	R	80%	R	85%	R	90%	R	95%	R	100%	R	105%	R	Vol	Dvol	Wvol	Mvol	Load	Dload	WkLoad	MoLoad	Sets	Dsets	WkSets	MoSets	WkAvi	MAvi
18	1	1	Snatch	78		85	1	91		98	1	104	1	111	1	117	1	124	1	130	2	137	2		11			1280.5				12	12				
18	1	2a	Clean	96	1	104	1	112	1	120	1	128	1	136	1	144	1	152	1	160	2	168	2		11			1576				12	12				
18	1	2b	Jerk	96	1	104	1	112	1	120	1	128	1	136	1	144	1	152	1	160	2	168	2		11			1576									
18	1	3	Snatch Extension	78		85		91		98		104		111		117		124		130	8	137	8		8			1040				4					
18	1	4	Front Squat	120	1	130	1	140		150		160	1	170	1	180	1	190		200	2	210	2		11	52		1970	7443			12	40				
18	2	1	Snatch	78	2	85	2	91	2	98	2	104	2	111	2	117	4	124		130		137			10			988				5					
18	2	2a	Clean	96	2	104	2	112	2	120	2	128	2	136	2	144	4	152		160		168			10			1216				5					
18	2	2b	Jerk	96	1	104	1	112	1	120	1	128	1	136	1	144	2	152		160		168			5			608									
18	2	3	Clean Extension	96		104		112		120		128		136		144		152		160	8	168			8			1216				4					
18	2	4	Good Morning	48		52		56		60		64		68		72		76		80	8	84	16		16	49		1280	5308			4	18				
18	3	1	Power Snatch	78	1	85	1	91	1	98	2	104	2	111	2	117		124		130		137			8			747.5				9					
18	3	2a	Power Clean	96	1	104	1	112	1	120	2	128	2	136	2	144		152		160		168			8			920				9					
18	3	2b	Jerk	96	1	104	1	112	1	120	2	128	2	136	2	144		152		160		168			8			920									
18	3	3	Back Squat	150	2	163	2	175		188	2	200	2	213	2	225	2	238	2	250	1	263			11			2162.5				6					
18	3	4	Press	48		52		56		60		64		68		72	12	76	12	80		84			12	47		864	5614			4	28				
18	5	1	Snatch	78	1	85	1	91		98	1	104	1	111	1	117	1	124	1	130	2	137	2		11			1280.5				12	12				
18	5	2a	Clean	96	1	104	1	112	1	120	1	128	1	136	1	144	1	152	1	160	2	168	2		11			1576				12	12				
18	5	2b	Jerk	96	1	104	1	112	1	120	1	128	1	136	1	144	1	152	1	160	2	168	2		11			1576									
18	5	3	Front Squat	120	1	130	1	140		150		160	1	170	1	180	1	190		200	2	210	2		11			1970				12					
18	5	4	Snatch Extension	78		85		91		98		104		111		117		124		130	8	137	8		8	52		1040	7443			4	40				
18	6	1	Power Snatch	78	1	85	1	91	1	98	2	104	2	111	2	117		124		130		137			8			747.5				9					
18	6	2a	Power Clean	96	1	104	1	112	1	120	2	128	2	136	2	144		152		160		168			8			920				9					
18	6	2b	Jerk	96	1	104	1	112	1	120	2	128	2	136	2	144		152		160		168			8			920									
18	6	3	Press	48		52		56		60		64		68		72	12	76	12	80		84		12	36	236		864	3452	29259		4	22	148			124.0

Table A.1 20-Week Program Excel Analysis: Week 18

Table A.1 20-Week Program Excel Analysis: Week 19

Wk	Day	Order	Exercise	60%	R	65%	R	70%	R	75%	R	80%	R	85%	R	90%	R	95%	R	100%	R	105%	R	Vol	Dvol	Wvol	Mvol	Load	Dload	WkLoad	MoLoad	Sets	Dsets	WkSets	MoSets	WkAvl	MAvl
19	1	1	Snatch	78		85		91		98	1	104	1	111	1	117	1	124	1	130	1	137	1	8				890.5				9					
19	1	2a	Clean	96	1	104	1	112	1	120	1	128	1	136	1	144	1	152	1	160	1	168	1	8				1096				9					
19	1	2b	Jerk	96	1	104	1	112	1	120	1	128	1	136	1	144	1	152	1	160	1	168	1	8				1096									
19	1	3	Front Squat	120	1	130		140	1	150	1	160	1	170	1	180	1	190	1	200	1	210	1	7	31			1160	4243			9	27				
19	2	1	Power Snatch	78	2	85		91	6	98	6	104	3	111		117		124		130		137		17				1501.5				10					
19	2	2a	Power Clean	96	2	104		112	6	120	6	128	3	136		144		152		160		168		17				1848				10					
19	2	2b	Jerk	96	1	104		112	3	120	3	128	3	136		144		152		160		168		10				1104									
19	2	3	Back Squat	150	3	163		175	3	188	3	200	3	213	3	225	9	238		250		263		18	62			3487.5	7941			6	26				
19	4	1	Snatch	78	1	85		91	1	98	1	104	1	111	1	117	2	124	1	130	1	137	1	6				611				6					
19	4	2a	Clean	96	1	104		112	1	120	1	128	1	136	1	144	2	152	1	160	1	168	1	6				752				6					
19	4	2b	Jerk	96	1	104		112	1	120	1	128	1	136	1	144	1	152	1	160	1	168	1	6				752									
19	4	3	Snatch Extension	78		85		91		98		104		111		117		124		130	8	137		8				1040				4					
19	4	4	Front Squat	120	2	130		140	2	150	2	160	2	170	2	180	2	190	4	200		210		12	38			1900	5055			6	22				
19	6	1	Snatch	78	2	85		91	2	98	2	104	2	111	2	117	2	124		130		137		8				767				4					
19	6	2a	Clean	96	2	104		112	2	120	2	128	2	136	2	144	2	152		160		168		8				944				4					
19	6	2b	Jerk	96	1	104		112	1	120	1	128	1	136	1	144	1	152		160		168		4				472									
19	6	3	Clean Extension	96		104		112		120		128		136		144	4	152		160		168		4				544				4					
19	6	4	Press	48		52		56		60		64		68		72		76		80		84		12	36	167		912	3639	20878		4	16	91			125.0

Wk	Day	Order	Exercise	60%	R	65%	R	70%	R	75%	R	80%	R	85%	R	90%	R	95%	R	100%	R	105%	R	Vol	Dvol	Wvol	Mvol	Load	Dload	WkLoad	MoLoad	Sets	Dsets	WkSets	MoSets	WkAvl	MAvl
20	1	1	Snatch	78	1	85		91		98	1	104	1	111	1	117	1	124		130		137		4				383.5				4					
20	1	2a	Clean	96		104	1	112		120	1	128		136	1	144	1	152		160		168		4				472				4					
20	1	2b	Jerk	96		104	1	112		120	1	128		136	1	144	1	152		160		168		4				472				4					
20	1	3	Front Squat	120		130	2	140		150	2	160		170	2	180	2	190		200		210		8				1180				4					
20	1	4	Press	48		52		56		60		64		68		72		76		80		84		12	32			912	3420			4	16				
20	2	1	Power Snatch	78		85	2	91		98	1	104		111		117		124		130		137		5				416				3					
20	2	2a	Power Clean	96		104	2	112		120	1	128		136		144		152		160		168		5				512				3					
20	2	2b	Jerk	96		104	1	112		120	1	128		136		144		152		160		168		3	13			312	1240			3	6				
20	3	1	Power Snatch	78		85	6	91		98		104		111		117		124		130		137		6				468				3					
20	3	2a	Power Clean	96		104	6	112		120		128		136		144		152		160		168		6				576				3					
20	3	2b	Jerk	96		104	3	112		120		128		136		144		152		160		168		3				288				3					
20	3	3	Jumping Back Squat	150	6	163		175		188		200		213		225		238		250		263		6	21	66	809	900	2232	6892	98216	3	9	31	427	104.4	121.4035847
			Macrocycle Total	1042		444		1665		236		1451		887		887		39		240		0					7782				910945				2321		117.06
			Macrocycle Percentages	0.134		0.057		0.214		0.030		0.186		0.114		0.114		0.005		0.031		0.031															40.965
						0.191				0.244				0.300				0.119																			
						19.10%				24.40%				30.00%				11.90%				3.10%															

Table A.1 20-Week Program Excel Analysis: Week 20

GRAPH INDEX

TABLE INDEX

REFERENCES

Ajan, T, Baroga, L. Weightlifting For All Sports. 1988

Baker, G. The United States Weightlifting Federation Coaching Manual Volume 3 Training Program Design. 1982

Bruner, R, Tabachnik, B. Soviet Training and Recovery Methods 151—243. 1990

Medvedyev, AS. A System of Multi-Year Training in Weightlifting. Translated by Andrew Charniga, Jr. 1989

Medvedyev, AS. A Program of Multi-Year Training in Weightlifting. Translated by Andrew Charniga, Jr. 1995.

Volgarev, MN, Korovnikov, KA, Valovaya, NI, Azizbekgan, GA. Essentials of Nutrition for Athletes. Soviet Sports Review Vol 22, No 4. 195—198. 1988.

Yessis, M. Secrets of Soviet Sports Fitness and Training. 151—182. 1987

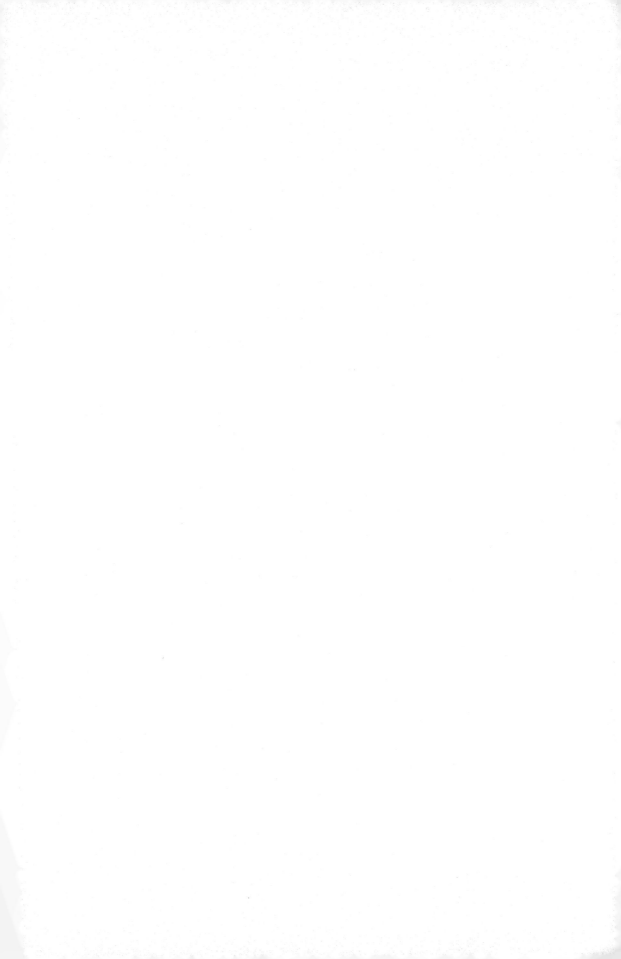

Made in the USA
Columbia, SC
10 July 2018